DIABETES AND TEA

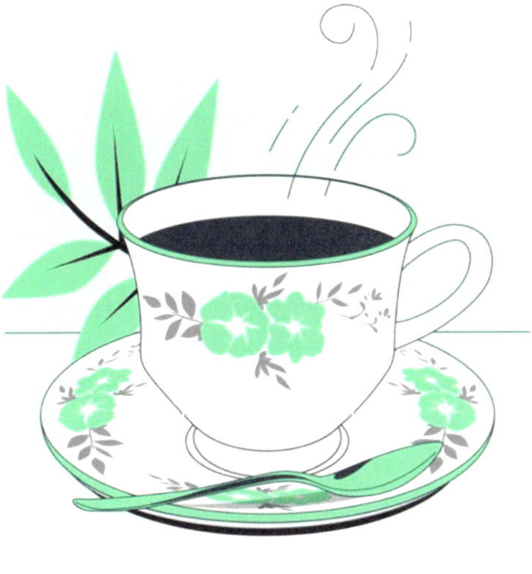

NASIM BELL
THE TEA LADY

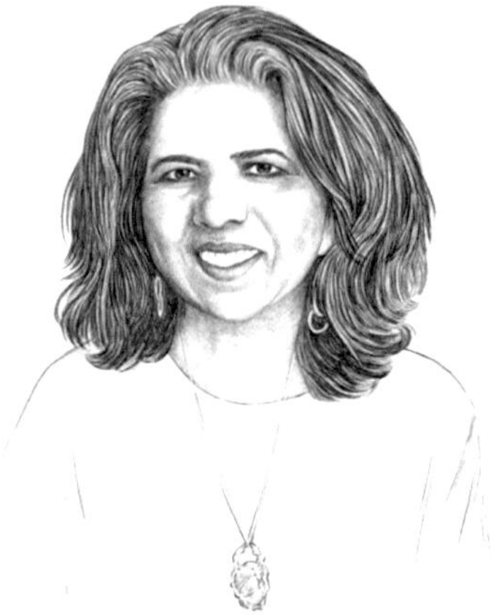

Nasim Bell - The Tea Lady

Nasim Bell, affectionately known as The Tea Lady, has spent over a decade immersed in the world of tea, studying its rich traditions, wellness benefits, and cultural significance. As the founder of Hummingbird Tearoom, she has cultivated a deep understanding of how tea can support overall health and well-being.

Through years of serving tea to customers from all walks of life, Nasim has had the privilege of hearing firsthand accounts of how tea has helped people manage their blood sugar levels. Many of her customers have shared inspiring stories of how incorporating tea into their daily routine has led to noticeable improvements in their health, helping to stabilize glucose levels, increase insulin sensitivity, and support overall metabolic balance.

Driven by these real-life experiences and her passion for natural wellness, Nasim set out to explore the science behind tea's role in diabetes management. In Diabetes and Tea, she blends centuries-old wisdom with modern research, offering readers a practical and approachable guide to harnessing the power of tea for blood sugar balance.

With a deep respect for nature and a commitment to helping others cultivate healthier habits, Nasim invites readers to discover how a simple cup of tea can be a powerful tool in their wellness journey.

It's Never Not Teatime®

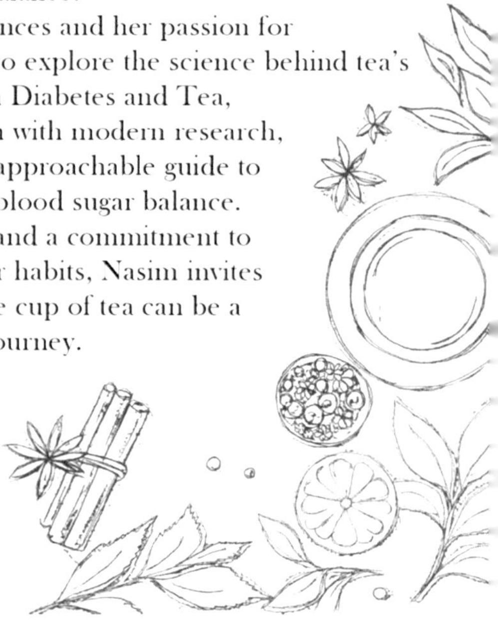

TABLE OF CONTENTS

INTRODUCTION: THE SWEET DILEMMA – CAN TEA REALLY HELP?

Diabetes is everywhere. You don't have to look far to see the impact—family, friends, neighbors, maybe even yourself. The numbers are staggering. Over the past few decades, diabetes has transformed from a rare condition to a global crisis.

Millions of people are living with it, and millions more are on the brink. Modern diets, stress, and sedentary lifestyles have all played a role in fueling this epidemic. Processed foods, hidden sugars, and an overreliance on convenience have become part of daily life, making it harder than ever to maintain stable blood sugar levels. And while there's no shortage of medications and medical advice, many people are left searching for something more—something natural, effective, and sustainable.

That's where tea comes in. Not as a magic bullet, not as a cure-all, but as a powerful, time-tested ally. Cultures around the world have relied on tea for centuries, not just as a comforting ritual but as a tool for wellness. From ancient Chinese medicine to Ayurvedic traditions in India, tea has been revered for its ability to support digestion, calm the mind, and promote overall balance in the body.

And now, science is catching up, confirming what traditional healers have known all along: certain teas contain compounds that may support blood sugar regulation, insulin function, and inflammation management when combined with a healthy lifestyle.

In Hummingbird Tearoom, we've had countless customers share their stories—some newly diagnosed, others managing diabetes for years—who have turned to tea as part of their wellness journey. Many of them are looking for simple, natural ways to support their health, and tea has become a gentle yet effective companion on that path.

They ask which teas might help curb sugar cravings, which ones promote better digestion, or which ones could provide steady energy without the spikes and crashes of sugary drinks. Time and time again, I've seen how even small changes, like swapping out sugary beverages for a thoughtfully chosen tea, can have a noticeable impact.

But let's be clear: this isn't about replacing medical treatment with a cup of tea. It's about adding another layer of support, another tool in the toolbox. The beauty of tea is its accessibility. It's simple, natural, and for most people, completely safe.

Unlike fad diets or extreme regimens, incorporating tea into your daily routine isn't drastic or difficult. It's a small, intentional step that can make a real difference over time. Even something as effortless as brewing a cup of cinnamon tea in the evening or sipping on green tea throughout the day can become a mindful, health-conscious habit.

This book is here to change the way you see tea. It's not just a beverage—it's a botanical powerhouse with real potential to support blood sugar balance. We'll dive into the science behind different types of teas, explore the specific compounds that make them effective, and offer practical ways to integrate them into your lifestyle. Whether you're looking for gentle support or a daily ritual to complement your existing routine, this book will give you the knowledge and confidence to make tea work for you.

So, can tea really help with diabetes? Let's find out.

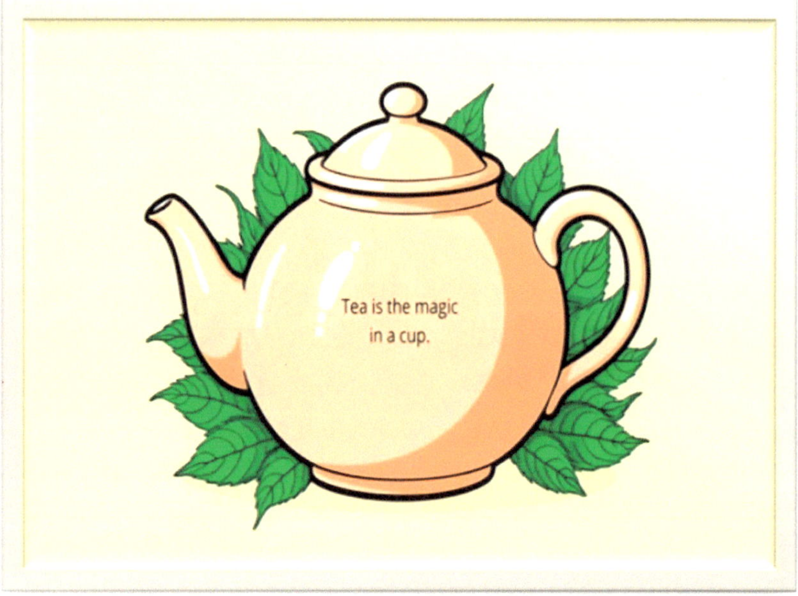
Tea is the magic
in a cup.

CHAPTER 1: THE SCIENCE OF BLOOD SUGAR – WHAT'S BREWING INSIDE YOUR BODY?

UNDERSTANDING BLOOD SUGAR SPIKES AND CRASHES

WHAT IS BLOOD SUGAR?

Blood sugar, or blood glucose, refers to the concentration of glucose circulating in your bloodstream. This glucose comes from the foods you eat, primarily carbohydrates, and serves as the primary source of energy for your body's cells. The regulation of blood sugar levels is a tightly controlled process, influenced by hormones, lifestyle choices, and dietary intake.

THE CYCLE OF BLOOD SUGAR SPIKES AND CRASHES

When you consume carbohydrates, your body breaks them down into glucose, which enters your bloodstream. The pancreas then releases insulin, a hormone that helps transport glucose into cells for energy or storage. However, this process doesn't always happen smoothly, leading to fluctuations in blood sugar levels, commonly known as spikes and crashes.

Blood Sugar Spikes:

A blood sugar spike occurs when glucose levels rise rapidly, often after consuming high-glycemic foods like refined sugars and processed carbohydrates. This can lead to:

- A burst of energy followed by a sharp drop.
- Increased production of insulin to move excess glucose into cells.
- Potential fat storage if glucose is not used for energy.
- Increased oxidative stress and inflammation.

Blood Sugar Crashes:

A crash happens when insulin overcompensates, causing blood sugar levels to drop too low, leading to:

- Fatigue and sluggishness.
- Increased hunger and sugar cravings.
- Mood swings and irritability.
- Brain fog and difficulty concentrating.

The Long-term Impact Of Blood Sugar Imbalance

Constant blood sugar fluctuations can increase the risk of insulin resistance, weight gain, metabolic disorders, and chronic diseases like type 2 diabetes and cardiovascular disease. Understanding how to balance blood sugar through diet, lifestyle, and mindful choices is essential for long-term health.

INSULIN RESISTANCE: THE SILENT DISRUPTOR

What Is Insulin Resistance?

Insulin resistance occurs when cells become less responsive to insulin, requiring more of the hormone to achieve the same glucose-lowering effect. Over time, the pancreas compensates by producing even more insulin, leading to chronically high levels of both insulin and blood sugar.

Causes Of Insulin Resistance

Several factors contribute to insulin resistance, including:

1. **Diet High in Refined Carbohydrates and Sugars:**
    - o Excess consumption of processed foods, sugary drinks, and refined grains can contribute to insulin resistance.
2. **Sedentary Lifestyle:**
    - o Lack of physical activity reduces the body's ability to regulate glucose effectively.
3. **Chronic Stress:**
    - o Elevated cortisol levels from stress can interfere with insulin signaling and blood sugar balance.
4. **Poor Sleep Patterns:**
    - o Inadequate sleep disrupts hormones that regulate blood sugar and increases cravings for high-carb foods.

5. **Excess Body Fat:**
    - o Particularly visceral fat around the abdomen, which releases inflammatory compounds that impair insulin function.

Signs And Symptoms Of Insulin Resistance

- Increased hunger and frequent cravings.
- Fatigue after meals.
- Difficulty losing weight, especially around the midsection.
- High fasting blood sugar levels.
- Darkened skin patches (acanthosis nigricans) around the neck, armpits, or groin.

The Progression From Insulin Resistance To Diabetes

If left unaddressed, insulin resistance can progress to prediabetes and eventually type 2 diabetes. This occurs when the pancreas can no longer keep up with the demand for insulin, leading to consistently high blood sugar levels. Early intervention through dietary modifications, exercise, and lifestyle changes can reverse insulin resistance and restore metabolic health.

THE ROLE OF ANTIOXIDANTS AND POLYPHENOLS IN METABOLIC HEALTH

What Are Antioxidants And Polyphenols?

Antioxidants are molecules that neutralize harmful free radicals in the body, reducing oxidative stress and inflammation. Polyphenols are a group of plant-based compounds with powerful antioxidant properties, found abundantly in tea, berries, cocoa, and various plant foods.

How Antioxidants Support Blood Sugar Regulation

Oxidative stress plays a significant role in insulin resistance and metabolic dysfunction. By combating oxidative damage, antioxidants help:

- Improve insulin sensitivity.
- Reduce inflammation.
- Protect pancreatic beta cells responsible for insulin production.
- Lower the risk of chronic diseases associated with high blood sugar levels.

THE POWER OF POLYPHENOLS

Polyphenols have been widely studied for their role in metabolic health, particularly in:

1. **Enhancing Insulin Sensitivity:**
    - Certain polyphenols, such as quercetin and resveratrol, improve the function of insulin receptors, making cells more responsive to insulin.
2. **Reducing Sugar Absorption:**
    - Polyphenols found in green tea, cinnamon, and bitter melon can slow the digestion of carbohydrates, leading to a more gradual rise in blood sugar levels.

3. **Decreasing Inflammation:**
    - o Chronic inflammation is a key contributor to insulin resistance. Polyphenols help reduce inflammatory markers, supporting metabolic health.

BEST DIETARY SOURCES OF POLYPHENOLS

Incorporating polyphenol-rich foods into your diet can have profound effects on blood sugar balance. Some of the best sources include:

- **Green Tea & Black Tea:** Rich in catechins and theaflavins, known for their blood sugar-lowering effects.
- **Berries (Blueberries, Strawberries, Blackberries):** Packed with anthocyanins that improve insulin sensitivity.
- **Dark Chocolate (70% Cocoa and Above):** Contains flavonoids that support glucose metabolism.
- **Cinnamon:** Contains polyphenols that mimic insulin and enhance glucose uptake by cells.
- **Turmeric:** The active compound curcumin has anti-inflammatory and blood sugar-regulating properties.
- **Olive Oil:** Contains hydroxytyrosol, a potent polyphenol that supports metabolic function.

Balancing Blood Sugar For Long-term Health

In my family, there was always a belief that maintaining stable blood sugar levels is key to overall well-being. By understanding the impact of blood sugar spikes and crashes, recognizing the dangers of insulin resistance, and incorporating antioxidant-rich foods into your diet, you can take control of your metabolic health.

Practical steps to support balanced blood sugar include:

- Eating a whole-food, nutrient-dense diet.
- Avoiding processed sugars and refined carbohydrates.
- Staying physically active and incorporating strength training.
- Managing stress through mindfulness, meditation, or deep breathing exercises.
- Getting sufficient quality sleep.
- Consuming antioxidant-rich foods and polyphenol-packed beverages like green tea.

By making these lifestyle changes, you can support your body's natural ability to regulate blood sugar, reduce the risk of metabolic diseases, and enjoy sustained energy levels throughout the day. The journey to balanced blood sugar starts with small, intentional choices that create long-lasting health benefits.

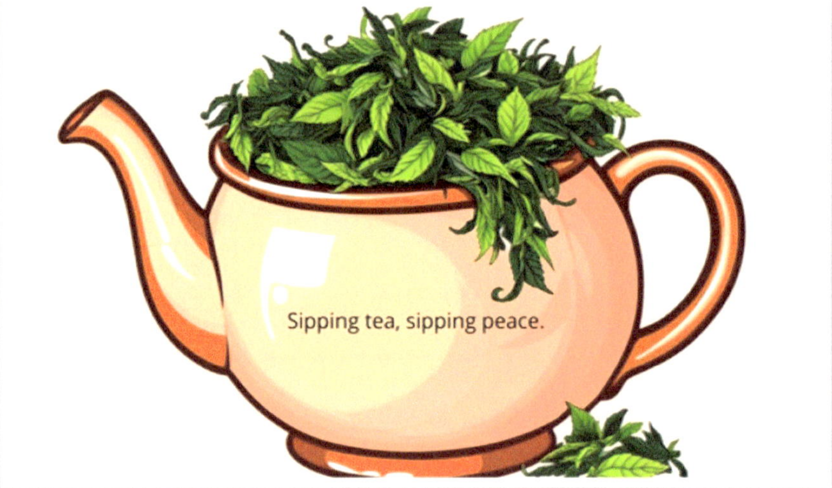
Sipping tea, sipping peace.

Chapter 2: How Tea Affects Blood Sugar – Sip By Sip Breakdown

The Magic Compounds: Catechins, Theaflavins, and Polyphenols

Picture this: You wake up groggy, shuffle into the kitchen, and put the kettle on. Maybe you reach for green tea, black tea, or even oolong. But as that warm cup meets your lips, something magical happens inside your body—a cascade of tiny compounds gets to work, some of which might be the key to keeping your blood sugar in check.

The star players here are catechins, theaflavins, and polyphenols. These aren't just fancy scientific words—these are the very molecules that make tea, well, tea. They give it its flavor, its color, and, most importantly, its ability to interact with our blood sugar levels.

- ### Catechins: Green Tea's Blood Sugar Whisperers

Catechins are abundant in green tea, and they're known for their antioxidant and anti-inflammatory properties. But what about blood sugar? In a 2016 study published in the *American Journal of Clinical Nutrition*, researchers found that catechins, particularly epigallocatechin gallate (EGCG), improved insulin function and reduced fasting blood sugar levels in participants with diabetes.

In simpler terms, catechins may help your body improve insulin efficiency, though effects can vary between individuals. Imagine your insulin is a key, and your cells are doors. Sometimes, with conditions like insulin resistance, those doors get jammed. Catechins act like a bit of WD-40, helping the key turn smoothly so glucose can enter the cells rather than staying outside in the bloodstream.

- THEAFLAVINS: BLACK TEA'S BOLD BENEFIT

If green tea has catechins, black tea has its own superstar: theaflavins. These polyphenols, formed during the oxidation of black tea leaves, are known for their deep amber color and strong taste. But their real magic happens inside the body. A 2021 study in *Scientific Reports* showed that black tea extract significantly reduced post-meal blood sugar spikes in participants with prediabetes.

Think of this as a buffer against sugar overload. When you eat something carb-heavy, theaflavins step in like traffic police, making sure sugar enters the bloodstream at a slower, more manageable pace.

- POLYPHENOLS: THE UNSUNG HEROES

All teas contain polyphenols, the broad family of antioxidants that fight inflammation, slow sugar absorption, and help insulin do its job. Studies from Harvard's School of Public Health confirm that polyphenols in tea can lower the risk of type 2 diabetes by improving glucose metabolism and reducing oxidative stress. These compounds essentially act like tiny personal trainers for your cells, keeping them fit and responsive to insulin.

CAFFEINE & METABOLISM: FRIEND OR FOE FOR DIABETICS?

Ah, caffeine. That beloved jolt of energy that gets us through mornings, late-night projects, and sluggish afternoons. But what does it do to blood sugar?

Here's where things get interesting. Caffeine's effect on metabolism is like a double-edged sword—it can help or hinder, depending on the person. Some studies, such as a 2018 review in the *Journal of Diabetes Research*, suggest that moderate caffeine intake can improve insulin sensitivity. Others, however, have found that excessive caffeine might temporarily increase blood sugar levels by triggering stress hormones like cortisol, which signals the liver to release more glucose into the bloodstream.

A Personal Experiment

A friend of mine, Raj, who has been managing type 2 diabetes for years, once did a little experiment. He drank a cup of strong black tea in the morning and tracked his blood sugar with a continuous glucose monitor. The result? A mild spike, but nothing dramatic. Then, he tried the same thing with coffee—his blood sugar shot up more noticeably. The reason? Coffee has a much higher caffeine content without the balancing polyphenols found in tea.

If you're diabetic or prediabetic, caffeine might be a trial-and-error situation. Some people find that it helps with metabolism and weight control, while others experience unwanted spikes. The trick is to listen to your body and test different teas to see how they affect you.

Insulin Sensitivity: Can Tea Really Make Cells Listen Better?

Imagine you're at a crowded party, trying to get someone's attention, but they just won't respond. That's kind of what happens in insulin resistance—your cells stop "listening" to insulin, making it harder for glucose to enter. The result? Higher blood sugar levels and a higher risk of diabetes complications.

Tea, however, might help.

A 2019 study in the *Journal of Nutrition &*

Metabolism found that habitual tea drinkers had significantly better insulin sensitivity compared to non-tea drinkers. The researchers credited this to tea's polyphenols, which help reduce inflammation and improve the function of insulin receptors.

This isn't just a lab discovery—many cultures have intuitively known this for centuries. In China, for example, drinking pu-erh tea after meals is a long-standing tradition believed to help digestion and regulate blood sugar. In Japan, matcha is consumed not just for its earthy taste but also for its metabolic benefits. And in India, spiced chai—often made with cinnamon, which has its own blood sugar-lowering properties—is a staple part of life.

Anecdotally, I've seen this work in my own family. My grandmother, who has mild insulin resistance, started drinking green tea daily a few years ago. Her blood sugar levels, which used to hover in the prediabetic range, stabilized within a few months. Was it just the tea? Maybe not entirely, but her doctor was impressed.

The Gut Connection: How Tea Influences Digestion And Sugar Absorption

Let's talk about your gut—because it turns out, it's more connected to blood sugar than most people realize.

Inside your digestive tract live trillions of bacteria, collectively known as the gut microbiome. These microbes play a role in breaking down food, absorbing nutrients, and even influencing blood sugar levels. Poor gut health can lead to inflammation, insulin resistance, and erratic glucose spikes.

Here's where tea comes in. A 2022 study in Gut Microbes found that tea polyphenols act as prebiotics, feeding good gut bacteria and improving the diversity of the microbiome. Healthier gut bacteria mean better digestion and steadier blood sugar control.

A Global Perspective

Different cultures have long used tea to aid digestion and blood sugar balance.

- In Morocco, sweetened mint tea is often sipped after meals. While the sugar content isn't ideal for diabetics, the mint itself can help with digestion and glucose regulation.
- In Russia, fermented tea like kombucha is popular, and some studies suggest that kombucha may help with glucose metabolism.
- In South America, yerba mate is traditionally consumed as an energy-boosting drink, but research shows it may also improve insulin function.

The key takeaway? Your gut is a major player in blood sugar regulation, and tea is one of the simplest (and tastiest) ways to support it.

Tea isn't a magic bullet, but it's certainly a powerful tool in the quest for balanced blood sugar. Whether it's green, black, oolong, or herbal, each sip carries compounds that work with your body in ways science is just beginning to understand. So, the next time you brew a cup, know that you're doing more than just enjoying a warm drink—you're giving your body a little extra support, sip by sip.

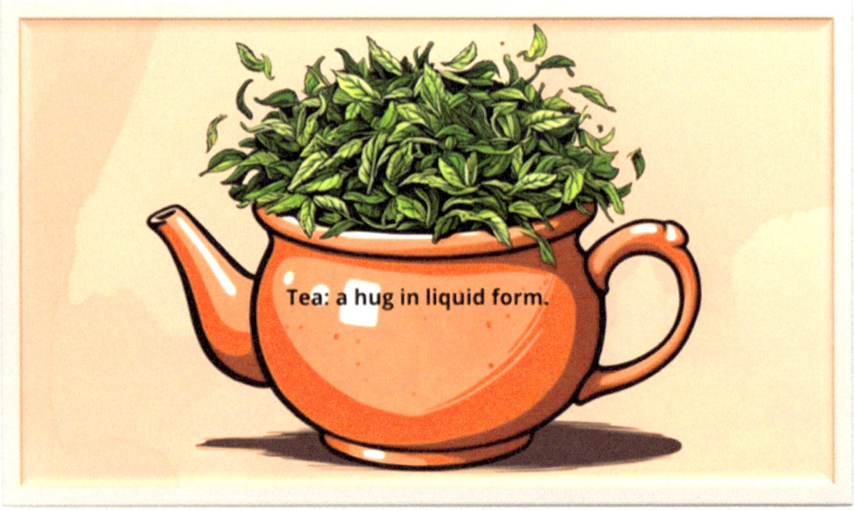
Tea: a hug in liquid form.

CHAPTER 3: FROM LEAF TO LIFELINE – THE BEST TEAS FOR DIABETES WARRIORS

A Deep Dive into Nature's Most Powerful Blood Sugar Regulators

Not all teas are created equal—especially when it comes to balancing blood sugar. Some teas work like gentle stabilizers, while others actively improve insulin sensitivity, reduce sugar absorption, and fight inflammation. In this chapter, we'll explore the best brews for diabetes warriors and how to make the most of them. Think of these teas as allies in your daily battle to regulate your blood sugar, transforming each sip into a small victory for your health.

1. Green Tea (Camellia sinensis) – The Metabolic Mastermind

Why EGCG (Epigallocatechin gallate) is a game-changer for glucose regulation:

Green tea is often hailed as one of the healthiest beverages on the planet, and for good reason. Packed with antioxidants, green tea's most celebrated compound, EGCG, plays a starring role in diabetes management. This potent antioxidant has been shown to help lower blood glucose levels by improving insulin sensitivity. EGCG works by stimulating the body's metabolism and improving glucose uptake by cells, reducing excess sugar in the bloodstream. If you're looking for a metabolic boost, green tea is a great starting point.

Studies linking green tea to better insulin function:

Scientific research has consistently supported green tea's role in improving insulin function. Numerous studies have shown that those who regularly consume green tea have better glucose control and insulin sensitivity compared to those who don't. In fact, some studies suggest that drinking green tea can reduce the risk of developing Type 2 diabetes. The evidence is mounting that this humble tea is a powerful ally for maintaining balanced blood sugar.

Best times to drink green tea for maximum impact:

Timing matters when it comes to green tea. For optimal blood sugar regulation, aim to drink it during meals or within 30 minutes after eating. The catechins in green tea help slow the absorption of carbohydrates, which can lead to a more gradual rise in blood sugar. Avoid drinking it too late in the day, though—it does contain caffeine, which may interfere with your sleep patterns. A morning or afternoon cup is ideal to enjoy both the health benefits and the mental clarity boost that comes with it.

2. Black Tea (Camellia sinensis) – The Underrated Hero

The theaflavins effect: How black tea slows down sugar absorption: Black tea might seem like a simple cup of comfort, but it's actually a powerhouse when it comes to managing blood sugar. Theaflavins, unique antioxidants found in black tea, have been shown to slow down the absorption of glucose in the digestive tract, which helps prevent blood sugar spikes after meals. These antioxidants act like slow-release mechanisms, allowing the body to process sugar more gradually rather than experiencing sharp spikes. In essence, black tea is like a shield for your blood sugar after every meal.

Does adding milk cancel out its benefits? (Spoiler: It depends!):

You may have heard that adding milk to black tea negates its health benefits, but the truth is a bit more nuanced. While some studies suggest that milk can reduce the bioavailability of antioxidants in tea, the effect is minimal when consumed in moderation. If you're concerned about maximizing the benefits of black tea, consider enjoying it without milk. But if you prefer your tea with a splash of dairy, don't stress—your body is still reaping many benefits.

Fermented vs. standard black tea: Which is better for diabetes?

Black tea comes in many forms, but when it comes to diabetes, fermented black tea—such as Pu-erh tea—might offer additional benefits. Fermented black tea has been shown to improve blood sugar regulation more effectively than standard black tea, thanks to its unique fermentation process that enhances the tea's antioxidant levels. If you're looking to add some variety to your tea collection, consider experimenting with a few cups of Pu-erh for its rich flavor and potential extra benefits for blood sugar control.

3. White Tea (Camellia sinensis) – The Gentle Insulin Whisperer

The least processed tea with the highest antioxidants:

White tea is the least processed of all teas, making it a rich source of antioxidants, including catechins and polyphenols. These powerful compounds help neutralize harmful free radicals in the body, which is particularly important for those with diabetes, as oxidative stress is a known contributor to blood sugar instability. White tea's delicate, smooth flavor is a great option for anyone looking to enjoy tea without the overpowering flavors of green or black tea.

How white tea fights oxidative stress, a major diabetes culprit:

Oxidative stress occurs when there's an imbalance between free radicals and antioxidants in the body. In diabetics, oxidative stress can accelerate complications such as nerve damage, kidney problems, and cardiovascular issues. White tea is packed with antioxidants that help reduce this oxidative damage, making it a gentle yet effective way to support long-term diabetes management.

A low-caffeine alternative to green tea with similar benefits:

If you're sensitive to caffeine or simply prefer a milder brew, white tea is an excellent alternative to green tea. It contains less caffeine, but it still delivers many of the same health benefits, including enhanced insulin sensitivity and reduced blood sugar levels. Whether you're looking for a late-night tea or simply a gentler alternative to green tea, white tea offers a subtle, soothing solution.

4. Oolong Tea (Camellia sinensis) – The Blood Sugar Stabilizer

The best of both worlds between green and black tea:

Oolong tea is like the perfect hybrid, offering a unique balance between green and black tea. It's partially fermented, which means it possesses some of the benefits of both types of tea.

Oolong has been shown to enhance fat metabolism and improve blood sugar control, making it a fantastic choice for those with diabetes who are looking to maintain stable glucose levels throughout the day.

How oolong tea reduces post-meal sugar spikes:

One of the key benefits of oolong tea is its ability to reduce post-meal blood sugar spikes. After eating, your body releases insulin to help absorb glucose into your cells. Oolong tea helps increase insulin sensitivity, allowing your body to process sugar more efficiently and preventing that dreaded spike in glucose levels after meals.

Best brewing method for diabetes-friendly oolong:

To extract the full benefits of oolong tea, it's important to brew it properly. Use water just below boiling (around 185°F to 200°F) to preserve the delicate flavors and nutrients. Steep it for about 3-5 minutes for the perfect cup. For diabetes management, drink it before or during meals to help mitigate sugar absorption and stabilize blood glucose levels.

5. Jiaogulan Tea – The Dual Support for Blood Sugar and Blood Pressure

A unique balance for metabolic health:

Jiaogulan tea, often called the "herb of immortality," is a powerful adaptogenic tea known for its ability to regulate both blood sugar and blood pressure. Rich in saponins, flavonoids, and antioxidants, it helps the body maintain metabolic balance while promoting overall cardiovascular health.

How Jiaogulan tea helps stabilize blood sugar and pressure:

Jiaogulan tea enhances insulin sensitivity, helping the body utilize glucose more effectively and reducing post-meal sugar spikes. This makes it a great choice for those managing diabetes or looking to prevent blood sugar fluctuations. Additionally, it supports healthy blood pressure by promoting nitric oxide production, which relaxes blood vessels and improves circulation, reducing strain on the heart.

Best brewing method for optimal benefits:

To get the most out of Jiaogulan tea, steep it in water around 185°F to 200°F for 3-5 minutes. This preserves its potent bioactive compounds. For blood sugar control, drink it before or during meals, and for blood pressure support, enjoy it throughout the day as a soothing, heart-friendly beverage.

6. Hibiscus Tea (Hibiscus sabdariffa) – The Pressure Regulator

A caffeine-free powerhouse for diabetics: Hibiscus tea is a vibrant, caffeine-free herbal brew that's packed with health benefits, especially for diabetics. Known for its striking red color, hibiscus tea has been shown to help regulate both blood sugar and blood pressure. For those looking to manage their diabetes without the stimulating effects of caffeine, hibiscus is the perfect option.

Double benefits: Balances blood sugar & lowers blood pressure:

Hibiscus tea offers a unique two-for-one benefit for people with diabetes. Not only does it help lower blood sugar, but it also has a reputation for regulating blood pressure. Both of these factors are crucial for overall heart health, which is especially important for diabetics, as they are at a higher risk of cardiovascular issues. By incorporating hibiscus into your routine, you're giving your body the tools it needs to stay balanced and healthy.

The secret behind its vivid red color and glucose-lowering effects:

The vivid red color of hibiscus tea comes from anthocyanins, the same antioxidants that give blueberries and other berries their rich hue. These antioxidants are responsible for the tea's ability to fight oxidative stress and lower blood sugar levels. Drinking hibiscus tea regularly can help protect your body from the harmful effects of high blood sugar while providing a refreshing, tangy flavor.

7. Bitter Melon Tea (Momordica charantia) – The “Natural Insulin”

Why this bitter fruit is a sweet deal for diabetics:

Bitter melon is a tropical fruit that has been used for centuries in traditional medicine as a remedy for diabetes. It's often referred to as the “natural insulin” because its compounds mimic the effects of insulin in the body. Studies suggest that bitter melon tea may support blood sugar control, though individual responses can differ. It should complement—not replace—medical guidance.

The bioactive compounds that mimic insulin:

Bitter melon contains bioactive compounds like charantin, which directly affects glucose metabolism in the body. These compounds act as insulin mimics, helping to lower blood sugar levels and reduce the need for additional insulin. Drinking bitter melon tea regularly can help diabetics maintain better control over their glucose levels, especially when combined with a healthy diet and lifestyle.

How to brew it for maximum potency:

To make bitter melon tea, you can use either fresh or dried bitter melon slices. Boil the slices for 10-15 minutes to extract their active compounds. The resulting tea has a strong, bitter taste, so consider adding a touch of honey or stevia to sweeten it if necessary. Drink it once or twice a day, ideally before meals, to help control blood sugar spikes.

8. Nettle Tea (Urtica dioica) – The Sugar Detoxifier

Helps the pancreas work more efficiently: Nettle tea is another herbal brew that works wonders for managing diabetes. Packed with nutrients like iron, calcium, and magnesium, nettle tea helps support overall health and wellness, while its anti-inflammatory properties aid in glucose regulation. It also helps the pancreas function more efficiently, which is crucial for diabetics since the pancreas is responsible for insulin production.

How nettle reduces inflammation & blood sugar fluctuations:

Inflammation is a significant factor in diabetes, often leading to insulin resistance and fluctuating blood sugar levels. Nettle tea works by reducing inflammation throughout the body, helping to stabilize blood sugar levels. Regular consumption of nettle tea can help prevent the inflammation that often accompanies uncontrolled diabetes.

A powerhouse of chromium & magnesium (key minerals for diabetes):

Chromium and magnesium are two essential minerals for diabetes management, and nettle tea is packed with both. Chromium helps improve insulin sensitivity, while magnesium plays a role in regulating blood sugar levels. By incorporating nettle tea into your routine, you're giving your body the tools it needs to manage blood sugar more effectively.

TEA & DIABETES: CULTURAL WISDOM FROM AROUND THE WORLD

For centuries, tea has been more than just a beverage—it has been a source of healing, tradition, and community. Across different cultures, tea plays an important role in health management, including blood sugar control. While modern science is only recently confirming what many traditional systems have long known, people from around the world have used tea as part of their approach to wellness and balance.

1. TRADITIONAL CHINESE MEDICINE (TCM) & TEA FOR BLOOD SUGAR

In Traditional Chinese Medicine (TCM), balance is key. High blood sugar is often linked to "**heat**" **and** "**dampness**" in the body, and certain teas are recommended to restore harmony.

- **Pu-erh Tea:** This fermented black tea is commonly consumed in China after meals to aid digestion and slow sugar absorption. Studies show that pu-erh can **improve insulin sensitivity** and help regulate glucose levels.
- **Goji Berry & Chrysanthemum Tea:** This floral and slightly sweet herbal tea is often used in TCM to support **liver health and eye health**, both of which are essential for people with diabetes.

2. AYURVEDA & INDIAN HERBAL TEAS

In India, **Ayurveda**, the ancient system of medicine, has long recognized the power of herbs to balance blood sugar. Many traditional diabetic-friendly teas originate from Ayurvedic practices.

- **Tulsi (Holy Basil) Tea:** Tulsi is known as an **adaptogen**, meaning it helps the body adapt to stress. Since stress can raise blood sugar, tulsi tea is often recommended to **stabilize glucose levels and improve insulin function**.
- **Cinnamon & Fenugreek Tea:** This spiced tea is often consumed after meals to **reduce post-meal glucose spikes**. Fenugreek seeds, in particular, contain soluble fiber that slows carbohydrate digestion.

3. MOROCCAN MINT TEA & BLOOD SUGAR CONTROL

In Morocco, mint tea is more than just a drink—it's a symbol of hospitality. However, the **traditional preparation includes large amounts of sugar**, which can be problematic for diabetics.

- **Diabetes-Friendly Version:** If you love mint tea, consider preparing it with fresh spearmint and green tea leaves but **skip the sugar** or replace it with a touch of **stevia or cinnamon** for natural sweetness.
- **Spearmint's Role in Insulin Sensitivity:** Research suggests that spearmint may improve **hormonal balance and glucose metabolism**, making it a good option for people with insulin resistance.

4. SOUTH AMERICA'S YERBA MATE & DIABETES PREVENTION

Yerba mate, a stimulating herbal tea from Argentina, Brazil, and Paraguay, has been linked to **better glucose metabolism and fat oxidation**.

- Studies indicate that yerba mate can **improve insulin sensitivity** and help with weight management, both of which are crucial for diabetics.
- However, it contains **caffeine**, so it should be consumed in moderation by people sensitive to stimulants.

5. AFRICA'S ROOIBOS TEA: A CAFFEINE-FREE BLOOD SUGAR ALLY

Rooibos tea, native to South Africa, is **naturally caffeine-free** and packed with antioxidants.

- It contains **aspalathin**, a rare polyphenol that has been shown to **reduce blood sugar levels and combat insulin resistance**.
- Unlike other teas, rooibos doesn't **interfere with iron absorption**, making it a great option for those managing both **diabetes and anemia**.

THE TAKEAWAY

Tea traditions from around the world reveal a deep connection between **nature and health**. While different cultures have developed their own unique approaches to tea and blood sugar management, they all share a common theme: **using natural ingredients in mindful ways to support well-being**.

As you explore the world of tea, consider integrating these cultural perspectives into your own diabetes management routine. Whether it's **a daily cup of green tea like in Japan, cinnamon-spiced chai like in India, or herbal rooibos from South Africa**, you can enjoy the best of tradition while making choices that support your health.

Diabetes Warrior Testimonial

Carlos' Journey: A Tea-Driven Approach to Blood Sugar Control

Carlos, a 54-year-old accountant from Texas, had always struggled with managing his blood sugar levels. Diagnosed with type 2 diabetes five years ago, he found himself constantly battling fatigue, sugar cravings, and fluctuating glucose levels despite following his doctor's recommendations. "I thought I was doing everything right—eating balanced meals and exercising—but my numbers were still unpredictable," he recalls.

One evening, while researching natural ways to support diabetes management, Carlos stumbled upon the potential benefits of green tea and cinnamon tea. Intrigued, he decided to swap his afternoon coffee for a cup of green tea and began drinking cinnamon tea before bed. Within weeks, he noticed subtle changes—fewer cravings, improved digestion, and more stable energy levels throughout the day.

After three months, his blood sugar readings became significantly more stable. His doctor was impressed. "Tea didn't replace my medication, but it became an essential part of my daily routine, making everything else work better." Today, Carlos continues his tea ritual and encourages others in his diabetes support group to explore the benefits of tea as part of a holistic approach to health.

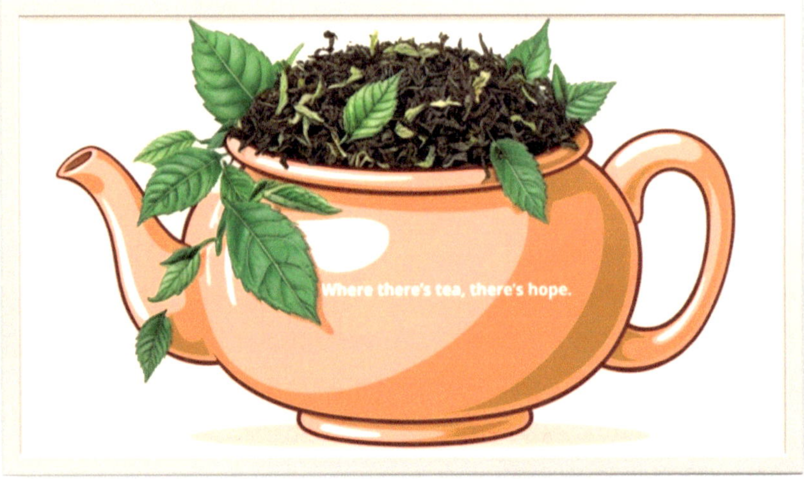
Where there's tea, there's hope.

CHAPTER 4: SUGAR & TEA – A LOVE STORY THAT NEEDS TO END?

Ah, sugar and tea. It's like the Romeo and Juliet of the beverage world: a love that's doomed from the start. We all know it's easy to pour a little sugar into our tea, especially when we're craving something sweet. But here's the thing: that sweet little habit might be doing more harm than good. So, let's take a step back and ask, should sugar and tea be in a relationship at all?

In this chapter, we're going to dive into the hidden dangers of sweetened tea, talk about why you should consider ditching sugar, and explore healthier, more fun ways to sweeten your brew. Plus, we'll chat about some sugar alternatives—like Stevia, monk fruit, and cinnamon—that could be your new best friends in the tea world.

Let's get started!

The Hidden Dangers Of Sweetened Tea

Okay, so we've all been there. A cup of tea sounds like the perfect pick-me-up. You boil the kettle, pour the hot water over your leaves (or tea bag, we're not judging), and then—bam! You add a spoonful of sugar. It's easy, it's comforting, and, let's face it, it tastes delicious. But here's the thing:

sugar doesn't just sit quietly in your tea, it's sneaky.

Every time you sweeten your tea, you're adding a little something extra to your body—something that might not be as sweet as you think. Sugar is a hidden culprit in many drinks, and it can sneak up on you like an unwelcome guest. Before you know it, you've consumed a chunk of your daily sugar intake in a single cup, and your body is none the wiser.

WHY IT'S NOT SO SWEET

Let's talk numbers for a second. A standard teaspoon of sugar has about 16 calories, and most people end up adding more than one to their cup of tea. If you're someone who drinks multiple cups of tea a day and sweetens them all, that sugar can add up quickly.

And we all know that sugar is a double-edged sword. On one hand, it gives you that quick energy boost. On the other hand, it can wreak havoc on your blood sugar levels, your waistline, and your overall health.

When you consistently drink sugary tea, you're essentially setting your body up for blood sugar roller coasters. First, you get a spike in energy—hello, sugar rush! But soon after, you're heading down the slope into a blood sugar crash. That crash? Not fun. You feel sluggish, irritable, and maybe even more tired than before. Plus, the long-term effects of sugar can be even worse. High sugar intake has been linked to an increased risk of heart disease, type 2 diabetes, and even certain cancers.

And let's not forget about weight gain. Sugar doesn't just sit around waiting to be used for energy—it gets stored as fat if your body doesn't need it right away. So, if you're sipping sweetened tea all day long, you might notice your jeans fitting a little tighter, even if you're not doing anything different in your diet. It's sneaky, remember?

THE EMOTIONAL ATTACHMENT

And don't even get me started on the emotional attachment we develop to sugar. Have you ever noticed how a sweetened cup of tea just feels like comfort? It's like you're drinking a hug.

Tea is one of those things that can feel incredibly soothing, and adding sugar makes it feel like an extra special treat. But here's the tough love part: That comfort comes at a price.

We get hooked on that sweetness, and suddenly, we're reaching for sugar every time we brew a cup. The more sugar we add, the more we crave, and before we know it, we're on a sugar high that's hard to shake. It's kind of like that relationship you know isn't good for you, but it's just so easy to keep going back to, right? Yeah, we've all been there.

So, how do we break up with sugar in our tea?

Healthier Ways To Sweeten Your Tea (without Spiking Blood Sugar)

Good news: You don't have to resign yourself to a bland cup of tea forever. There are plenty of ways to sweeten your tea without bringing sugar into the picture. And you'll still get that delightful sweetness without the guilt. Let's explore some healthier options that won't send your blood sugar on a rollercoaster ride.

1. TRY HONEY—IN MODERATION

Honey is a classic choice, and it's definitely a step up from refined sugar. Why? Because honey contains natural sugars like glucose and fructose, which your body processes a bit differently. Plus, it's packed with antioxidants and has anti-inflammatory properties. So, when you add a little honey to your tea, you're not just sweetening it, you're also adding some health benefits.

But—and this is a big but—moderation is key. Even though honey is a more natural sweetener, it's still sugar. Too much honey can still cause blood sugar spikes. Stick to a small drizzle, and you'll be good to go.

2. MAPLE SYRUP—NATURE'S LIQUID GOLD

If you're a fan of the maple syrup flavor (who isn't?), then it's time to consider adding a splash to your tea. Like honey, maple syrup has a more complex flavor profile, and it also contains minerals like manganese and zinc. These are good for your immune system and bone health, making maple syrup a fun and flavorful way to sweeten your tea without the usual sugar rush.

Again, use it sparingly. A little maple syrup goes a long way in adding both sweetness and flavor.

3. COCONUT SUGAR—FOR A SUBTLE, CARAMEL-LIKE TASTE

If you like a deeper, almost caramel-like sweetness in your tea, coconut sugar might just be your new best friend. It's made from the sap of coconut palms and retains a lot of the natural nutrients found in the coconut. Coconut sugar contains iron, zinc, calcium, and potassium, as well as some antioxidants. It's not a miracle worker, but it's certainly a healthier alternative to refined sugar.

One perk of coconut sugar is that it has a lower glycemic index than regular sugar, which means it won't cause as dramatic a spike in blood sugar levels. Still, don't go overboard—it's still sugar.

4. AGAVE NECTAR—SWEET, BUT NOT OVERPOWERING

Agave nectar is another alternative that has gained popularity in recent years, and for good reason. It's sweeter than sugar, so you need less of it. It has a very low glycemic index, meaning it won't cause rapid spikes in blood sugar. Plus, it dissolves easily in both hot and cold beverages, making it a great choice for iced teas.

That said, agave nectar is also high in fructose, which can cause issues if consumed in large amounts. So, as with all sweeteners, moderation is important.

5. FRUIT INFUSIONS—NATURE'S CANDY

One of the healthiest (and most natural) ways to sweeten your tea is by infusing it with fruit. Think berries, citrus, or even apples. You can steep fruit directly in your tea or even mash it up and add it to the brew. Not only does this add a natural sweetness, but it also gives your tea an extra burst of vitamins and antioxidants.

Try adding slices of lemon or orange to your green or black tea for a refreshing twist. Or throw in some berries for a fruity punch that will naturally sweeten your cup.

STEVIA, MONK FRUIT, AND CINNAMON – THE BEST ALTERNATIVES

So, we've talked about some more natural sweeteners, but what if you want something that's really low on the sugar scale? Stevia, monk fruit, and cinnamon are all excellent alternatives for those looking to reduce sugar intake while still getting that sweet taste.

1. STEVIA – THE PLANT-BASED SWEETENER THAT WON'T SPIKE BLOOD SUGAR

Stevia is derived from the leaves of the Stevia rebaudiana plant, and it's way sweeter than sugar. A little goes a long way with stevia, so you don't need to use much to get a sweet taste. The best part? Stevia has zero calories and doesn't raise your blood sugar levels, making it a perfect choice for diabetics and anyone watching their sugar intake.

Some people find stevia a little too sweet or get an aftertaste they don't love, but if you can handle it, stevia is a fantastic option for sweetening tea without any of the sugar-related downsides.

2. MONK FRUIT – THE SWEETNESS WITHOUT THE GUILT

Monk fruit (Siraitia grosvenorii) is another natural sweetener that has taken the health world by storm. Unlike sugar, monk fruit doesn't raise blood sugar levels and has zero calories. It's extracted from the monk fruit plant, and it's about 150-200 times sweeter than sugar, so you only need a small amount to sweeten your tea.

Monk fruit is a great option for those who want the sweetness of sugar without the crash or the health risks. Plus, it doesn't have the funky aftertaste that some people dislike about stevia.

3. CINNAMON – THE SWEET SPICE WITH EXTRA BENEFITS

Cinnamon is more than just a delicious spice to sprinkle on your oatmeal. It can also be used as a natural sweetener in your tea! While cinnamon doesn't taste sweet in the traditional sense, it has a natural ability to enhance the sweetness of other flavors. Plus, cinnamon itself has been shown to help regulate blood sugar levels, so it's a win-win. Add a cinnamon stick to your tea or sprinkle a little ground cinnamon in your cup to give it that cozy sweetness without the sugar spike.

Natural Sweeteners & Their Effects

Sweetener	Glycemic Index	Pros	Cons
Sugar	65	Provides quick energy	Causes rapid blood sugar spikes
Honey		Contains antioxidants	Still raises blood sugar
Maple Syrup	54	Rich in minerals	Should be used in moderation
Agave Nectar	15	Low glycemic index	High in fructose, can affect metabolism
Stevia	0	Zero calories, no impact on blood sugar	Some people dislike the aftertaste
Monk Fruit	0	Natural and antioxidant-rich	Can be expensive
Cinnamon	0	May help lower blood sugar	Works best as an addition, not a primary sweetener

TIME TO BREAK UP WITH SUGAR

So, there you have it. It's time to break up with sugar in your tea—there are so many better options out there. Whether you go for honey, maple syrup, or one of the natural alternatives like stevia, monk fruit, or cinnamon, you can enjoy a delicious, sweetened cup of tea without the health risks that sugar brings.

By ditching sugar and opting for healthier alternatives, you'll be doing your body a big favor. You'll avoid the blood sugar rollercoaster, keep your waistline happy, and maybe even feel a little bit better overall. So, the next time you reach for your tea bag, think about how you want to sweeten it—and make the choice that's best for you.

Let's say goodbye to the sugar rush and hello to a new chapter in your tea journey! Cheers!

Tea time, me
time.

CHAPTER 5: THE RITUAL OF TEA – HOW DRINKING MINDFULLY IMPROVES HEALTH

MORE THAN A DRINK: THE DEEP ROOTS OF TEA CULTURE

Tea is not just something people drink. It's a rhythm, a habit, a silent companion to life's most ordinary and extraordinary moments. It carries the weight of history, of generations who have found comfort in its warmth, of rituals that stretch back centuries.

Some people measure time in years, others in seasons. But in many cultures, time is marked by the number of cups poured, the way the leaves unfurl, the scent that lingers in the air.

For me, tea is deeply personal. It's woven into my family's heritage, tied to India, where my parents are from, and Zambia, where I was born. Tea in Zambia, much like in India, is not a rushed affair. It's not something you gulp down on your way out the door, distracted by notifications and the demands of the day. It's something you make time for, something that gathers people together.

Mornings in our home began with a steaming cup of chai—strong black tea infused with spices like cardamom, ginger, and cloves, simmered with milk until it reached just the right depth of flavor. The aroma alone was enough to signal the start of the day. Even in Zambia, where English-style tea traditions are common, my family held onto the Indian way of preparing and enjoying tea.

Beyond chai, there were other traditions too. Rooibos, native to South Africa, found its way into many Zambian households, appreciated for its earthy sweetness and deep red hue. Some drank it plain, others with a splash of honey or a squeeze of lemon. And in the rural areas, where life is still closely connected to the land, fresh lemongrass was often plucked and steeped in hot water, filling kitchens with its bright, citrusy scent.

But Zambia and India are not the only places where tea is more than just a drink. Tea has carved its place in cultures across the world, each one adding its own layer of meaning, its own method of preparation, its own belief in the quiet power of a well-brewed cup.

A World United By Tea, A World Divided By Preparation

Step into a tea house in Japan, and you won't just be given a cup of tea—you will witness an entire performance. The Japanese tea ceremony, or **chanoyu**, is a practice rooted in Zen Buddhism, where every movement is deliberate, every action infused with mindfulness.

The tea master doesn't simply make tea; they guide participants through an experience of presence and simplicity. The bowl is turned just so, the whisking of the matcha is precise, and even the act of drinking is done with full attention.

Now, contrast this with Morocco. Here, tea is bold, theatrical. Moroccan mint tea is not simply poured—it is lifted high, the stream cascading into delicate glasses, the foam forming at the top a sign of a skilled pour. It's an offering, a way of saying, "You are welcome here." The tea itself—green tea blended with fresh spearmint and generous amounts of sugar—is both invigorating and sweet, a drink meant to be sipped while conversations stretch long into the evening.

Then, there's China, where tea is ancient, diverse, and deeply ingrained in daily life. The **gongfu cha** method is an intricate practice where tea is steeped multiple times in small clay pots, each infusion revealing new depths of flavor.

Pu-erh tea, a fermented variety, is prized not just for its taste but for its supposed digestive and health benefits, something that Chinese medicine has long advocated.

In India, tea is about spice and warmth. Chai is not just tea; it's an experience. Black tea is simmered with milk, infused with ginger, cardamom, cloves, cinnamon, and pepper, creating a drink that is both soothing and stimulating. Vendors—**chaiwalas**—serve it in tiny clay cups on the streets, the scent of spices mingling with the hum of daily life.

From Turkish **çay** served in tulip-shaped glasses to Russia's **samovar** culture, where tea is kept hot all day long, every corner of the world has found its own way of honoring tea. Yet, across all these cultures, one thing remains the same: tea is a ritual, a moment of pause, a reason to gather.

Tea And The Science Of Health: How Tradition Meets Modern Medicine

For centuries, people have trusted tea for more than just comfort. Healers, shamans, and herbalists have turned to tea as medicine, using it to soothe digestion, calm the nerves, and fight illness. But now, science is starting to explain what traditional cultures have long known: tea isn't just good for the soul—it's good for the body.

One of the most exciting areas of research is tea's role in **blood sugar regulation and diabetes management**. This is something my grandmother seemed to know instinctively, even without scientific studies.

She would drink strong, unsweetened bush tea and say it kept her "balanced." At the time, I didn't think much of it. But today, researchers have found that certain teas, particularly green, black, and rooibos, contain powerful compounds that can help regulate glucose levels.

- **Green Tea and Blood Sugar:** Green tea is rich in **catechins**, antioxidants that improve insulin sensitivity and reduce inflammation. Studies show that regular green tea drinkers tend to have lower fasting blood sugar levels and a reduced risk of developing type 2 diabetes.
- **Black Tea's Hidden Power:** Black tea, the very same tea my family drinks daily in Zimbabwe, contains **theaflavins**, which have been shown to slow the absorption of sugar into the bloodstream, preventing dangerous spikes.
- **Rooibos and Aspalathin:** Rooibos tea, a caffeine-free herbal tea from southern Africa, contains a rare antioxidant called **aspalathin**, which research suggests may improve insulin resistance and help maintain stable blood sugar levels.

Beyond diabetes, tea has been linked to heart health, weight management, and even improved mental clarity. The **L-theanine** in green and black tea helps induce a calm yet focused state of mind, explaining why monks in China and Japan have long used tea as a meditation aid.

But while the science is fascinating, the way we drink tea matters just as much as the tea itself.

The Art Of Drinking Tea Mindfully

Tea isn't meant to be rushed. Unlike coffee, which is often gulped down in a hurry, tea asks us to slow down. The process of making tea—heating the water, measuring the leaves, waiting for the infusion—forces us to be present.

Mindful tea drinking is not a new concept. The Japanese have practiced it for centuries. The British have built entire social customs around it. Even in Zimbabwe, where tea is often enjoyed during family gatherings or quiet mornings, there is an unspoken rule: tea is not to be rushed.

Science backs this up. Studies on mindful eating and drinking suggest that being fully present with what we consume improves digestion, reduces stress, and even helps regulate metabolism. When we drink tea mindfully, we engage our senses—the warmth of the cup, the aroma of the leaves, the way the liquid feels as we swallow. This simple act can be a form of meditation, a way to anchor ourselves in the present moment.

So, the next time you make a cup of tea, take a breath. Notice the color of the liquid, the scent rising with the steam. Hold the cup in your hands and feel its warmth. Take a slow sip and pay attention to the way it moves across your tongue.

In a world that is always rushing, let tea be your reminder to pause.

Because tea is not just a drink. It's a ritual. It's history in a cup. It's connection—to the past, to others, to yourself. And in that connection lies its greatest power.

A Morning Tea Ritual for Blood Sugar Balance

Start your day with intention and a balanced blood sugar level by incorporating this simple yet effective tea ritual into your morning routine.

1. **Wake Up and Hydrate:** Begin with a glass of room-temperature water with a splash of lemon to kickstart digestion and hydration.
2. **Choose Your Tea:**
    - **Green tea (for metabolism and insulin sensitivity)**
    - **Cinnamon tea (to help lower blood sugar levels)**
    - **Ginger tea (for anti-inflammatory and digestive benefits)**
3. **Mindful Brewing:**
    - Heat water to **160-180°F** (for green tea) or **boiling** (for herbal teas).
    - Steep for **3-5 minutes** for optimal nutrient extraction.

    - While steeping, take deep breaths and set an intention for the day.
4. **Enhance Naturally:**
    - Add a pinch of **cinnamon** or **turmeric** for additional blood sugar benefits.
    - Use **stevia** or **monk fruit** instead of sugar if you prefer sweetness.
5. **Sip Slowly & Engage Your Senses:**
    - Take small sips and enjoy the aroma.
    - Feel the warmth, appreciate the flavors, and start your day with a moment of mindfulness.

By integrating this ritual, you set a foundation for balanced energy levels and better blood sugar control throughout the day.

Simple 5-minute Tea Meditation (to Reduce Sugar Cravings & Stress)

1. **Hold the cup in both hands.** Feel the warmth.
2. **Close your eyes and breathe deeply.** Inhale through your nose, exhale slowly.
3. **Focus on the aroma.** What notes do you smell—floral, earthy, spicy?
4. **Take a slow sip.** Notice how the tea moves across your tongue.
5. **Express gratitude.** Thank yourself for making time to care for your health.

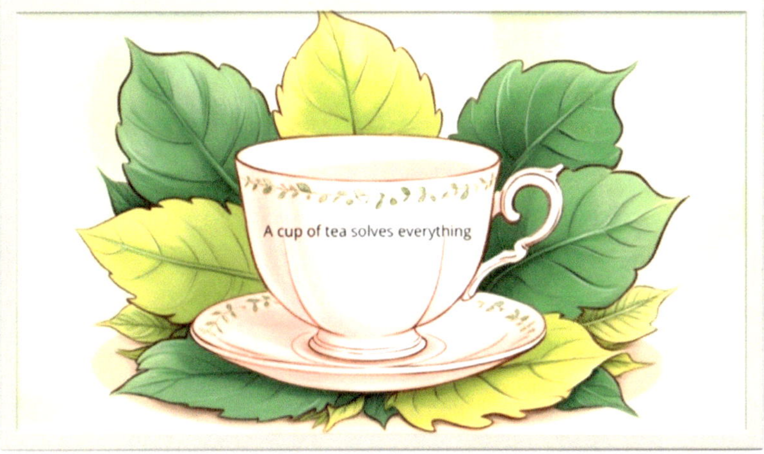
A cup of tea solves everything

CHAPTER 6: TEA ALCHEMY – CRAFTING THE PERFECT BLEND FOR BLOOD SUGAR BALANCE

HOW TO MIX, MATCH & CUSTOMIZE YOUR OWN DIABETES-FRIENDLY TEA BLENDS

I. The Art & Science Of Tea Blending

If you've ever thought that managing blood sugar means boring diets and avoiding all the good stuff, think again. Tea is one of those small, daily rituals that can actually help keep your glucose levels in check—*if* you know how to blend the right ingredients.

Single-ingredient teas, like cinnamon or ginger, are powerful on their own. But when combined, teas can work in harmony to create an even stronger effect on blood sugar balance. Think of it like assembling a dream team: each ingredient brings its own superpower, but together, they're unbeatable.

A great diabetes-friendly tea blend has three key components:

1. **Blood Sugar Regulators** – Herbs that actively lower glucose levels.
2. **Metabolic Boosters** – Ingredients that improve insulin sensitivity and help the body process sugar better.

3. **Nutrient Enhancers** – Plants that replenish essential minerals and antioxidants often depleted in people managing diabetes.

Now, let's dive into these categories and see how you can build the ultimate tea blend for blood sugar control.

II. BUILDING BLOCKS: KEY INGREDIENTS FOR A POTENT ANTI-DIABETES TEA BLEND

BLOOD SUGAR REGULATORS – THE FOUNDATION OF YOUR BLEND

These are the heavy hitters when it comes to stabilizing glucose levels.

- **Cinnamon Bark (Cinnamomum verum)** – Not only does cinnamon add warmth and spice to your tea, but studies suggest it can slow digestion and lower fasting glucose levels. Research even shows it mimics insulin, making it a must-have for any anti-diabetes tea blend.
- **Mulberry Leaf (Morus alba)** – A star in traditional Chinese medicine, mulberry leaf prevents sugar spikes after meals by blocking carbohydrate absorption in the gut. Think of it as your natural glucose traffic cop.
- **Bilberry Leaf (Vaccinium myrtillus)** – A cousin of the blueberry, bilberry leaves

support insulin production and can help keep blood sugar levels steady. Plus, they add a slightly fruity note to your tea.

- **Ivy Gourd (Coccinia grandis)** – Used in Ayurveda for centuries, this plant mimics insulin activity and can reduce post-meal blood sugar spikes.
- **Purslane (Portulaca oleracea)** – A surprising but potent ingredient, purslane is packed with alpha-linolenic acid, an essential fatty acid linked to better glucose metabolism.

METABOLIC BOOSTERS – ENHANCING INSULIN SENSITIVITY

These ingredients help your body use insulin more efficiently, reducing resistance and improving blood sugar response.

- **Moringa Leaf (Moringa oleifera)** – Moringa is a powerhouse of nutrients and antioxidants that fights inflammation, which is a key factor in insulin resistance.
- **Holy Basil (Ocimum tenuiflorum)** – Stress raises blood sugar, and holy basil is known for lowering cortisol levels. Less stress, fewer sugar spikes!
- **Lemon Peel (Citrus limon)** – A zesty addition to your tea, lemon peel is rich in

polyphenols that reduce oxidative stress linked to diabetes.

- **Ginger Root (Zingiber officinale)** – Not just for nausea! Ginger improves gut health, which plays a huge role in insulin sensitivity.

NUTRIENT ENHANCERS – REPLENISHING VITAL MINERALS FOR DIABETIC HEALTH

Many people managing diabetes experience deficiencies in key mi

nerals. These herbs help replenish them while offering additional blood sugar benefits.

- **Nettle (Urtica dioica)** – High in chromium and magnesium, nettle is excellent for regulating blood sugar levels naturally.
- **Hibiscus (Hibiscus sabdariffa)** – Aside from being beautifully tart and vibrant, hibiscus is loaded with vitamin C, which helps protect blood vessels from damage caused by high glucose levels.
- **Dandelion Root (Taraxacum officinale)** – This underrated ingredient supports liver detoxification, which is crucial for overall metabolic health.

III. DIY TEA BLENDS: FORMULAS FOR SPECIFIC NEEDS

Now, let's put these ingredients to work in practical, easy-to-make blends:

THE MORNING BLOOD SUGAR STABILIZER – FOR ENERGY WITHOUT A GLUCOSE SPIKE

- **Green Tea + Cinnamon + Ginger + Lemon Peel**
- Green tea adds antioxidants, cinnamon stabilizes glucose, ginger improves digestion, and lemon peel keeps stress-induced sugar spikes at bay.

THE POST-MEAL SUGAR SHIELD – TO PREVENT SPIKES AFTER EATING

- **Mulberry Leaf + Bilberry Leaf + Hibiscus + Moringa**
- Mulberry and bilberry regulate sugar absorption, hibiscus supports circulation, and moringa adds a metabolic boost.

THE NIGHTTIME BLOOD SUGAR SOOTHER – FOR BETTER SLEEP AND GLUCOSE CONTROL

- **Holy Basil + Rooibos + Chamomile + Nettle**
- Holy basil and chamomile calm the nervous system, while rooibos and nettle nourish the body with essential minerals.

THE DIGESTIVE BOOSTER – FOR PEOPLE WITH DIABETES-RELATED BLOATING OR SLUGGISH DIGESTION

- **Dandelion Root + Ginger + Lemon Peel + Fennel**
- A gut-friendly blend that promotes better digestion and nutrient absorption.

IV. THE RITUAL OF TEA – WHY PREPARATION MATTERS

Brewing tea is more than just dunking a bag in hot water. Here's how to do it right:

- **Infusions (for leaves and flowers)** – Steep for **5-10 minutes** in **hot but not boiling** water (around 175°F / 80°C). This method is great for delicate herbs like hibiscus and mulberry leaf.
- **Decoctions (for roots and barks)** – Simmer for **15-20 minutes** to extract the maximum benefits. Cinnamon and dandelion root need this treatment to release their full potential.

THE IMPACT OF ADDITIVES

- **Honey?** Use in moderation, as it can still spike blood sugar.
- **Lemon?** Yes! It enhances antioxidant absorption.
- **Milk?** Skip it. Dairy can interfere with some polyphenols in tea.

COLD BREW VS. HOT TEA – WHICH ONE IS BETTER FOR DIABETES?

Cold

brewing extracts fewer tannins, making it gentler on the stomach and less likely to spike blood sugar. It's a great option for summer or if you find hot tea too strong.

V. FINAL THOUGHTS: FINDING YOUR SIGNATURE BLEND

The best tea for you is the one that fits your unique needs. Start experimenting with different ingredients, listen to your body, and adjust your blends over time. Maybe you need a little more cinnamon or a touch of ginger—it's all about personalization.

Making tea a daily ritual doesn't just support blood sugar control—it turns a simple habit into a moment of mindfulness and self-care. So grab your teapot, start blending, and enjoy the process!

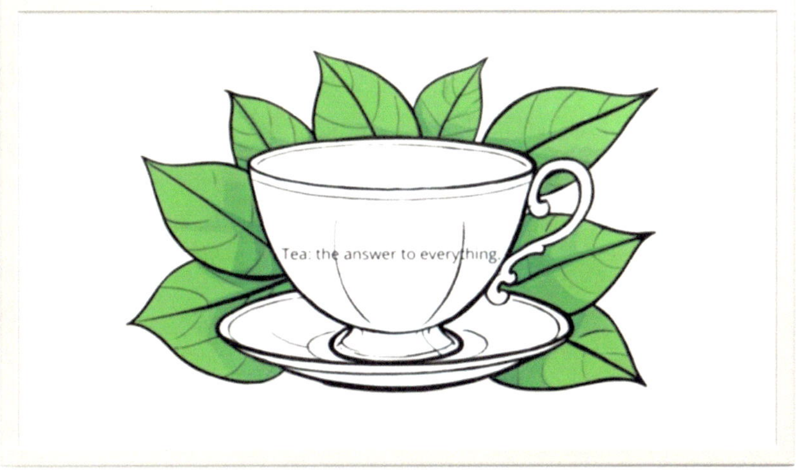
Tea: the answer to everything.

CHAPTER 7: BREWING FOR BALANCE – THE BEST WAYS TO PREPARE TEA FOR MAXIMUM BENEFITS

Now that we've explored the different types of tea and their benefits, it's time to focus on how to prepare them correctly. Brewing tea isn't just about dunking a tea bag into hot water and hoping for the best. The way you brew your tea can make or break its flavor and effectiveness. Get it right, and you'll extract all the soothing, energizing, or healing properties each variety has to offer. Get it wrong, and you might end up with something that tastes like disappointment.

So, how do we brew tea *correctly*—not just to avoid disasters, but to actually maximize its benefits? The answer is part science, part art, and a little bit of knowing when to let your tea do its thing. Let's break it down.

THE RIGHT TEMPERATURE AND STEEPING TIME FOR DIFFERENT TEAS

First things first—temperature and time matter. You wouldn't cook all foods at the same heat, right? (Imagine grilling a steak and baking a cake in the same oven at 500°F—absolute chaos.) Tea is the same. Here's a simple breakdown:

- **Green Tea:** 160-180°F (70-80°C)
    - o Anything hotter, and your tea turns into a mouthful of regret.
    - o Example: Ever had green tea that tasted like boiled spinach? Yeah, that was scalded.
- **Black Tea:** 200-212°F (93-100°C)
    - o This tea *wants* to be hot. Just don't overdo it unless you enjoy drinking astringency incarnate.
- **Oolong Tea:** 180-200°F (82-93°C)
    - o Think of it as the middle child of teas—neither too delicate nor too bold.
- **White Tea:** 160-185°F (70-85°C)
    - o It's the diva of teas—gently coax out its flavors or risk making it taste like hot water.
- **Herbal Tea:** 200-212°F (93-100°C)
    - o Since herbs aren't technically "tea" (gasp!), they need longer steeping to release their goodness.

Steeping time is often seen as a key factor in determining a tea's flavor and quality. However, in my tearoom experience, I found that shorter steeping times consistently produced the best results. We never brewed any tea or tisane for more than three minutes.

This approach resulted in a smooth, flavorful cup without the bitterness that can come from over-steeping. By keeping the steeping time brief, we also eliminated the need for sweeteners, allowing the tea's natural flavors and delicate nuances to take center stage.

Letting tea steep for a shorter time enables it to speak for itself. This method enhances the subtle taste profiles, making teas more approachable—especially for those who find strong or astringent flavors overwhelming. It also challenges traditional brewing guidelines, which can sometimes lead to an overly intense or inconsistent cup.

My friend once boiled water in a kettle, poured it straight over a bag of chamomile, and let it sit for 20 minutes. By the time she drank it, she described the taste as "like licking the bottom of a dusty flowerpot." Don't be like her. Follow the time guides.

HOT BREW VS. COLD BREW: DOES IT CHANGE THE BENEFITS?

Cold brewing tea sounds like something fancy and complicated, but it's actually the easiest method out there. Just integrate tea leaves into cold water, let them sit in the fridge overnight, and *bam*—smooth, refreshing tea. But does it offer the same benefits?

HOT BREW PROS:

- Extracts more antioxidants quickly (especially from green and black teas).

- Feels comforting (perfect for curling up with a book and pretending you have your life together).
- Releases bold, rich flavors.

COLD BREW PROS:

- Less bitter (because it extracts fewer tannins, which are responsible for that puckering astringency).
- Retains delicate flavors and certain heat-sensitive compounds.
- Lower caffeine content (it extracts more slowly, so it's great if you want less buzz).

When should you go cold?

- If you love smooth, naturally sweet tea.
- If you don't want to mess around with precise temperatures.
- If it's hot outside and the thought of a steaming mug makes you want to scream.

When should you go hot?

- If you need a strong, antioxidant-packed cup ASAP.
- If it's freezing outside and you want to feel alive again.
- If you're brewing something like ginger tea, where heat helps release its spicy kick.

Real-life example: One summer, I left a jar of oolong tea steeping in cold water overnight. The next day, it tasted like pure, floral bliss with zero bitterness. The only downside? I drank a whole liter without realizing it, which resulted in a slightly embarrassing caffeine buzz at a morning meeting.

Quick-Cold Tea

At the tearoom, making iced tea was never complicated—we always started with hot water. Steeping the tea in hot water first allows the flavors to fully develop before chilling it down. Once properly steeped, we strained the tea and poured it over ice, instantly cooling it while locking in the perfect taste.

The key to great iced tea isn't longer steeping times—it's using more tea. A stronger brew ensures the flavors remain bold and balanced even after the ice melts. Whether black, green, or herbal, this method guarantees a refreshing, full-bodied iced tea every time.

ADDING SPICES: HOW TURMERIC, BLACK PEPPER, AND CLOVES ENHANCE EFFECTS

Sure, tea is great on its own, but sometimes, it needs a little *something extra*. Enter spices—the superheroes of brewing. Not only do they add flavor, but they also supercharge the health benefits of your tea.

TURMERIC + BLACK PEPPER = ANTI-INFLAMMATORY POWER COUPLE

Turmeric is amazing, but here's the catch: your body doesn't absorb it well on its own. Black pepper, however, contains **piperine**, which boosts turmeric absorption by up to 2000%. (Yes, you read that right.)

How to Use It: Add a pinch of turmeric and a dash of black pepper to hot tea, especially chai or herbal blends. You can also add a little honey to balance the earthiness.

Real-life example: I once made a turmeric tea without pepper and wondered why it wasn't doing much. A week later, I added pepper, and suddenly, my joints felt happier, and I had a weirdly nice glow. Coincidence? I think not.

CLOVES – THE TINY BUT MIGHTY IMMUNE BOOSTER

Cloves are packed with antioxidants and have antimicrobial properties. They also give a spicy warmth to tea, making them perfect for winter blends.

How to Use It:

- Drop one or two whole cloves into your tea while it steeps.
- Try them in black tea, chai, or even ginger tea for extra depth.

Real-life example: I added too many cloves once and felt like I had brewed a cup of liquid Christmas potpourri. Lesson learned: less is more.

FINAL THOUGHTS: BREWING AS A RITUAL

At the end of the day, brewing tea isn't just about extracting the "right" compounds—it's about enjoying the process. Take a moment to appreciate the aroma, the warmth of the cup, the way the flavors unfold. Whether you're steeping a traditional green tea at precisely 175°F or adding a handful of herbs into a pot like a medieval alchemist, remember: it's your tea. Make it how *you* love it.

And if all else fails? **JUST DON'T MICROWAVE YOUR TEA.** Some rules are non-negotiable.

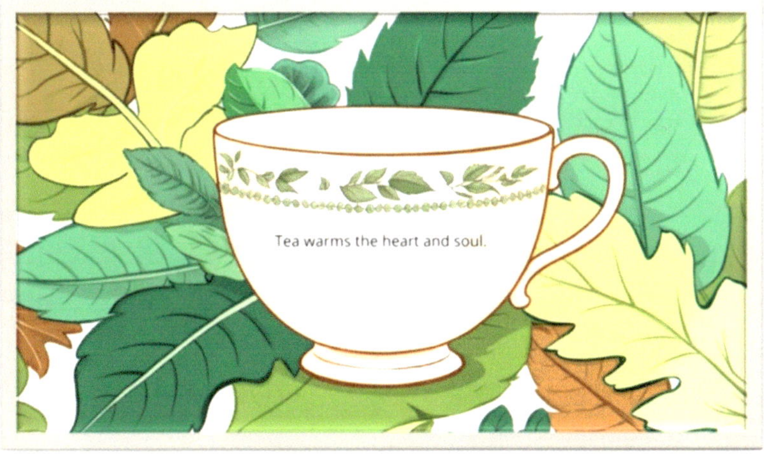
Tea warms the heart and soul.

CHAPTER 8: WHEN TEA BECOMES A PROBLEM – SIDE EFFECTS & PRECAUTIONS

We've spent a lot of time talking about the wonders of tea—its soothing qualities, its impressive health benefits, and the many ways you can prepare it to maximize those perks. But what happens when tea turns from a friend into a frenemy? Yes, it's possible.

Like anything else, tea isn't perfect, and while it offers a wealth of benefits, it also comes with a few warnings. If you've ever had a jittery caffeine overload, found yourself running to the bathroom after one too many cups, or wondered whether tea was messing with your iron levels, this chapter is for you. Let's get into the nitty-gritty of when tea becomes a problem and what you can do to enjoy it responsibly.

CAFFEINE SENSITIVITY: WHEN TOO MUCH TEA CAUSES MORE HARM THAN GOOD

Ah, caffeine—the reason many of us function in the morning. Tea has less caffeine than coffee, sure, but that doesn't mean it's harmless. Some teas, especially black and matcha, can pack quite a punch. If you're sensitive to caffeine, even a seemingly innocent cup of green tea in the evening might turn into a sleepless night filled with regrets.

Signs You've Had Too Much Tea:

- Jitters, anxiety, or that unsettling feeling that you could hear colors.
- A racing heart (your body's way of saying, "Hey, maybe slow down there").
- Insomnia, even when you *swore* that green tea wouldn't keep you up.
- Digestive issues—caffeine stimulates the gut, sometimes *too much*.

WHAT YOU CAN DO:

- **Switch to low-caffeine or caffeine-free teas.** Herbal teas like chamomile, rooibos, or peppermint are great options.
- **Try decaffeinated tea.** It's not entirely caffeine-free, but it's much gentler.
- **Watch your steeping time.** The longer you steep, the more caffeine gets extracted.

Real-life example: A friend once drank four cups of matcha before a big meeting, thinking it would help with focus. Instead, he spent the entire presentation gripping his chair like he was holding onto a rocket launch. Lesson? Moderation is key.

MEDICATION INTERACTIONS: CAN TEA INTERFERE WITH DIABETES DRUGS?

Tea is often praised for its ability to help regulate

blood sugar, but if you're on medication for diabetes, you'll want to be cautious. Some compounds in tea can either enhance or inhibit drug effectiveness.

WHAT'S THE ISSUE?

- **Green tea and diabetes medications:** Green tea can lower blood sugar levels, which *sounds* great, but when combined with medication that does the same thing, it could lead to *hypoglycemia*—low blood sugar.
- **Black tea and blood pressure meds:** Black tea contains compounds that can slightly raise blood pressure, potentially interfering with antihypertensive drugs.

WHAT YOU CAN DO:

- Talk to your doctor if you drink tea regularly and take medication.
- Space out tea consumption from medication time—give it at least an hour.
- Monitor your blood sugar levels if you're adding more tea to your routine.

Real-life example: My aunt, who has type 2 diabetes, started drinking three cups of green tea daily because she heard it was good for blood sugar control. One day, her glucose levels dropped too low, and she felt lightheaded. Her doctor adjusted her medication and recommended keeping tea consumption moderate.

IRON ABSORPTION & TEA: SHOULD YOU DRINK TEA BEFORE OR AFTER MEALS?

There's a long-standing debate about whether tea interferes with iron absorption, and science says: *yes, it does*—but only in certain cases.

How Tea Affects Iron Absorption

Tea contains tannins, which bind to iron from plant-based foods (non-heme iron) and make it harder for your body to absorb it. If you're vegetarian or prone to anemia, you *might* want to reconsider when you drink your tea.

WHAT YOU CAN DO:

- **Drink tea between meals, not with meals.** This reduces interference with iron absorption.
- **Pair iron-rich foods with vitamin C.** A splash of lemon juice in your tea can help counteract the tannins.
- **If you eat meat, you're fine.** Heme iron (from animal sources) isn't affected as much.

Real-life example: A friend who's a lifelong vegetarian always felt exhausted. After a blood test revealed low iron levels, her doctor suggested adjusting her tea-drinking habits. She started drinking tea between meals instead of during, added more vitamin C to her diet, and her energy levels improved.

THE DEHYDRATION MYTH: DOES TEA REALLY DEHYDRATE YOU?

For years, people have been told that tea dehydrates you because it contains caffeine. But is this actually true?

THE TRUTH:

- Yes, caffeine has a mild diuretic effect (meaning it makes you pee more), but the amount in tea is low enough that it doesn't *really* dehydrate you.
- If you drink tea in normal amounts, it still contributes to your daily fluid intake.
- However, if you drink a *lot* of highly caffeinated tea without balancing it with water, you might notice increased bathroom trips and mild dehydration symptoms.

WHAT YOU CAN DO:

- **Drink water alongside your tea.** It's an easy fix.
- **Avoid excessive caffeine intake.** If you're drinking six cups of black tea a day, maybe dial it back.
- **Opt for herbal teas.** No caffeine, no dehydration worries.

Real-life example: Someone I know tried a "tea detox" where they drank only tea for a whole day. By the evening, they felt tired, had a headache, and realized they hadn't had any actual water all day. Turns out, tea is great, but your body still needs good old-fashioned H_2O.

FINAL THOUGHTS: DRINK TEA, BUT KNOW YOUR LIMITS

Tea is an amazing beverage with countless benefits, but like anything else, it's best enjoyed in balance. Whether you're watching your caffeine intake, managing a medical condition, or just trying to make sure you're absorbing enough iron, a little awareness goes a long way.

At the end of the day, tea should make you *feel* good—not jittery, exhausted, or lightheaded. Pay attention to how your body reacts, make adjustments as needed, and enjoy your cup with confidence. And if all else fails? Switch to herbal. They never betray you.

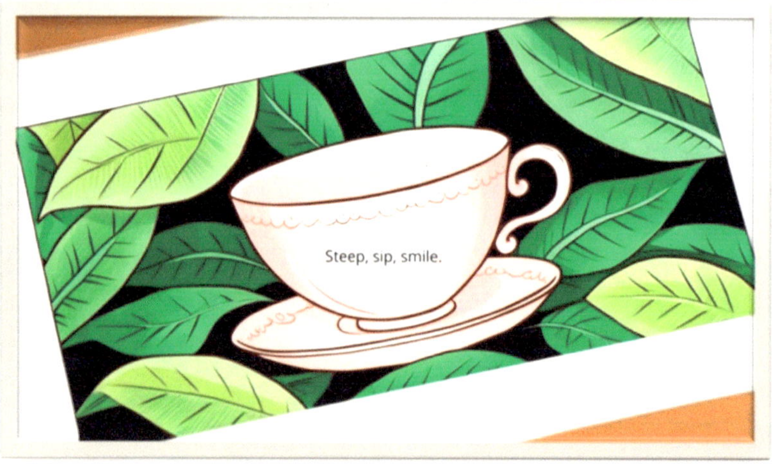
Steep, sip, smile.

CHAPTER 9: TEA VS. COFFEE – WHICH ONE WINS FOR DIABETES?

Ah, the great debate—tea versus coffee. It's a rivalry as old as time (or at least as old as your local coffee shop and tea house). If you're managing diabetes, you've probably wondered which drink is the better option.

Does one spike your blood sugar more than the other? Does caffeine play a sneaky role in insulin resistance? And most importantly—can you still enjoy both without wrecking your glucose levels? Let's break it down.

THE CAFFEINE CONUNDRUM: WHICH DRINK AFFECTS BLOOD SUGAR MORE?

Caffeine is the fuel that keeps many of us going, but its effects on blood sugar can be a little… complicated. Both coffee and tea contain caffeine, but in different amounts, and your body doesn't necessarily react to them the same way.

WHAT WE KNOW:

- **Coffee contains more caffeine than tea.** A standard 8-ounce cup of coffee has about 95 mg of caffeine, whereas black tea has around 47 mg, and green tea has even less at about 30 mg.

- **Caffeine can temporarily increase blood sugar.** Studies have shown that caffeine can cause a short-term rise in blood glucose levels by making cells more resistant to insulin. (*Source: American Diabetes Association*)
- **Long-term, caffeine may improve insulin sensitivity.** While caffeine might cause a temporary rise in blood sugar, some research suggests that habitual coffee or tea drinkers may develop improved insulin sensitivity over time. (*Source: Harvard T.H. Chan School of Public Health*)

So, what does this mean? If you drink coffee or tea occasionally, you *might* see a short-term glucose spike. But if you're a regular consumer, your body may adapt, and the long-term effects could actually be beneficial.

HOW COFFEE INTERACTS WITH INSULIN LEVELS

Coffee has a more complex relationship with insulin than you'd think. On one hand, some studies suggest that regular coffee consumption may lower the risk of developing type 2 diabetes.

On the other hand, caffeine itself can temporarily increase insulin resistance, meaning your body has to work harder to regulate blood sugar after drinking it.

WHAT'S HAPPENING?

1. **Caffeine blocks adenosine.** This is a neurotransmitter that influences insulin sensitivity. When caffeine blocks it, insulin resistance temporarily increases.
2. **Chlorogenic acid to the rescue.** Coffee contains chlorogenic acid, a powerful antioxidant that may help slow glucose absorption and improve insulin function in the long run.
3. **Decaf vs. regular.** Some research suggests that decaf coffee offers the same long-term benefits without the short-term blood sugar spike. (*Source: Journal of Nutrition & Metabolism*)

WHAT YOU CAN DO:

- If you notice blood sugar spikes after coffee, try **decaf** or **smaller servings**.
- Pair coffee with **a meal rich in fiber and protein** to reduce blood sugar fluctuations.
- Opt for **black coffee** or use low-glycemic sweeteners instead of sugar-heavy creamers.

TEA FOR THE WIN? UNDERSTANDING TEA'S EFFECT ON BLOOD SUGAR

Tea doesn't just offer a gentler caffeine boost—it also contains natural compounds that may help regulate blood sugar. Polyphenols, catechins, and theaflavins found in tea have been studied for their potential benefits in diabetes management.

WHAT MAKES TEA A GOOD CHOICE?

- **Green tea has been linked to improved insulin sensitivity.** The catechins in green tea, especially EGCG (epigallocatechin gallate), have been shown to help the body use insulin more effectively. (*Source: Diabetes & Metabolism Journal*)
- **Black tea may slow carbohydrate absorption.** Theaflavins in black tea can help moderate post-meal blood sugar spikes by slowing down digestion. (*Source: Journal of Agricultural and Food Chemistry*)
- **Herbal teas offer caffeine-free benefits.** Cinnamon tea, for example, has been studied for its ability to lower fasting blood sugar levels.

WHAT YOU CAN DO:

- **Drink green or black tea regularly** for potential long-term benefits.
- **Avoid adding sugar**—or try cinnamon or a splash of lemon for natural flavor.
- **Try herbal teas** like cinnamon or fenugreek if you want caffeine-free blood sugar support.

CAN YOU DRINK BOTH? FINDING THE RIGHT BALANCE

If you love both tea and coffee, the good news is—you don't necessarily have to pick a side. The key is to be mindful of your personal response to caffeine and adjust accordingly.

BEST PRACTICES FOR COFFEE AND TEA LOVERS WITH DIABETES:

- **Monitor your blood sugar.** Everyone reacts differently, so track your levels to see how coffee and tea affect you.
- **Stick to moderation.** One or two cups of coffee or tea per day is usually fine. Overloading on caffeine can lead to insulin resistance.
- **Drink tea in the evening.** If caffeine affects your sleep (which can impact blood sugar control), switch to tea in the afternoon or evening.
- **Consider decaf coffee.** If coffee is causing blood sugar spikes, decaf may still offer benefits without the caffeine-related drawbacks.

FINAL VERDICT:

- If you need **a gentler caffeine option** that supports blood sugar control, **tea is your best bet**.

- If you love coffee but worry about insulin resistance, **try decaf or pair it with fiber-rich meals**.
- If you want the best of both worlds, **enjoy them in moderation and pay attention to how your body reacts**.

At the end of the day, the winner isn't coffee or tea—it's *you*, making informed choices that keep your blood sugar steady while still enjoying your favorite beverages. So, whether you're sipping on a bold espresso or a soothing green tea, just remember: balance is everything.

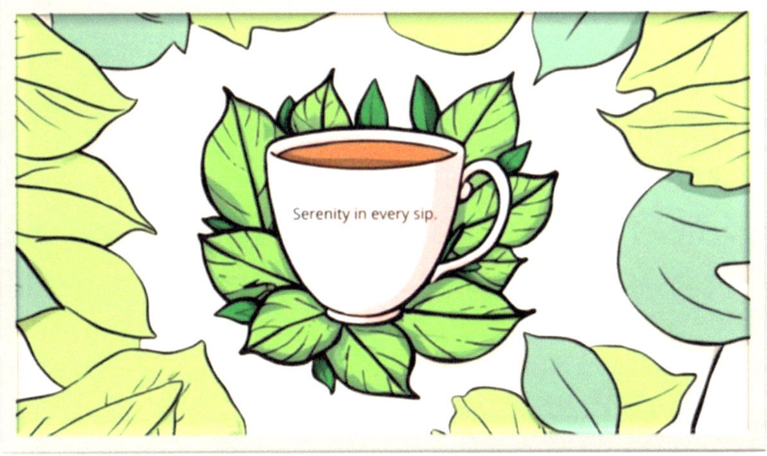
Serenity in every sip.

CHAPTER 10: STEEPING HOPE: HOW TEA HELPS PEOPLE MANAGE DIABETES ACROSS CULTURES

There is something deeply human about the way we seek healing in familiar places—through the rituals of our ancestors, the plants that grow around us, and the wisdom passed down in quiet conversations over steaming cups. For many, managing diabetes isn't just about following a doctor's orders; it's about finding a rhythm that feels natural, sustainable, and connected to something bigger than themselves.

Tea has long been woven into cultural traditions, not just as a drink but as a form of care. Some turn to it because their grandparents did. Others embrace it after modern science confirms what their ancestors already knew.

Whether it's bitter melon tea in the Philippines, mint tea in Morocco, or guava leaf tea in Mexico, these stories reveal the intimate ways people across the world blend tradition with personal health.

The following testimonials are not about replacing medicine but about reclaiming balance—one warm, deliberate sip at a time.

MARIA'S JOURNEY: BITTER MELON TEA IN THE PHILIPPINES

Growing up in a small fishing village in the Philippines, Maria watched her grandmother prepare *ampalaya* (bitter melon) tea every morning. "My *lola* swore by it," Maria recalls. "She always said it was our family's secret to staying strong."

When Maria was diagnosed with type 2 diabetes in her early fifties, she remembered her grandmother's advice. "At first, I was skeptical," she admits. "The taste is... well, bitter!" But after drinking one cup daily for three months, alongside her prescribed medication and a healthier diet, she noticed her blood sugar levels stabilizing.

In Filipino culture, *ampalaya* is widely used as both food and medicine, often recommended for its blood sugar-lowering properties. Modern studies have supported these claims, showing that bitter melon contains compounds that mimic insulin and help cells absorb glucose more efficiently. For Maria, this tea has become more than just a remedy—it's a connection to her heritage. "Every sip reminds me of my *lola* and the wisdom she passed down."

ABDUL'S TRADITION: CINNAMON-INFUSED MINT TEA IN MOROCCO

For Abdul, a retired artisan from Fez, Morocco, tea has always been a part of life. "In our culture, tea is sacred," he says. "It's how we welcome guests, how we relax, and even how we heal." Moroccan tea, typically a strong black tea infused with fresh mint, is a daily ritual.

After his diabetes diagnosis, Abdul's doctor advised him to reduce sugar intake, which meant cutting back on the traditional heavily sweetened Moroccan mint tea. Instead, he turned to cinnamon-infused black tea, an alternative his grandmother once recommended for digestive and blood sugar control. "At first, it was strange to drink tea without sugar," he admits. "But the cinnamon added a natural sweetness and warmth."

Cinnamon has long been used in Middle Eastern and North African medicine for its ability to improve insulin sensitivity. Recent research supports its potential role in lowering fasting blood sugar levels. Now, Abdul swears by his spiced tea, enjoying it twice a day. "It's comforting, healthy, and keeps my glucose levels in check—what more could I ask for?"

Anaya's Ayurvedic Wisdom: Tulsi Tea In India

For Anaya, an Ayurvedic practitioner from Kerala, India, the connection between tea and diabetes is deeply rooted in traditional Indian medicine. "Ayurveda has always emphasized the power of herbs, and tulsi, or holy basil, is one of our greatest gifts," she explains.

Anaya was diagnosed with prediabetes in her early thirties, a wake-up call that led her to explore her own healing traditions more deeply.

She began drinking tulsi tea twice a day, believing in its ability to reduce stress, improve metabolism, and support pancreatic function. "In Ayurveda, we see diabetes as an imbalance in the body," she says. "Tulsi helps restore that balance."

Scientific studies have highlighted tulsi's role in lowering blood glucose levels and improving overall health by reducing oxidative stress. Anaya now recommends it to many of her clients. "It's not a magic cure," she warns, "but it's a powerful ally."

JORGE'S FAMILY REMEDY: GUAVA LEAF TEA IN MEXICO

Jorge, a schoolteacher from Mexico City, remembers his mother brewing guava leaf tea whenever someone in the family fell ill. "She believed it could fix everything," he laughs. "Colds, stomach issues, even cuts and wounds—she always had a reason to make us drink it."

When Jorge was diagnosed with type 2 diabetes at 45, his mother reminded him of guava leaf tea's potential to lower blood sugar. Skeptical but willing to try, he began drinking a cup after meals. "To my surprise, my post-meal sugar spikes became much more manageable," he says.

Guava leaves contain compounds that slow carbohydrate absorption, helping to prevent sudden glucose surges. In Mexico, where diabetes rates are high, many families still turn to traditional herbal remedies alongside modern medicine. "I still take my prescribed medication," Jorge emphasizes, "but this tea is part of my daily routine now. It's like my mom is still looking out for me."

Eleanor's Love For Blueberry Leaf Tea In Canada

Eleanor, a retired nurse from Nova Scotia, grew up picking wild blueberries in the summer. "I always knew blueberries were good for you," she says, "but I never thought their leaves would be just as powerful."

After being diagnosed with diabetes, Eleanor came across an old Indigenous remedy—blueberry leaf tea. "The Mi'kmaq people have used it for generations to help with blood sugar," she explains. She started drinking it regularly and soon noticed an improvement in her energy levels and glucose readings.

Blueberry leaves contain antioxidants that enhance insulin function and reduce inflammation, making them a valuable herbal remedy. "It's amazing how nature provides for us," Eleanor reflects. "Sometimes, the answers have been right in front of us all along."

Conclusion: A Shared Tradition Of Healing

These testimonials, spanning different cultures and traditions, highlight the universal connection between tea and healing. While no tea is a standalone cure for diabetes, many people have found comfort and support in their traditional herbal remedies.

Whether it's bitter melon in the Philippines, cinnamon tea in Morocco, tulsi in India, guava leaves in Mexico, or blueberry leaf tea in Canada, each culture offers its own wisdom—steeped in history and hope.

For those managing diabetes, integrating these teas alongside medical advice, a balanced diet, and exercise can provide additional support. Most importantly, these teas connect people to their heritage, reminding them that healing is not just about science—it's about tradition, family, and the wisdom passed down through generations.

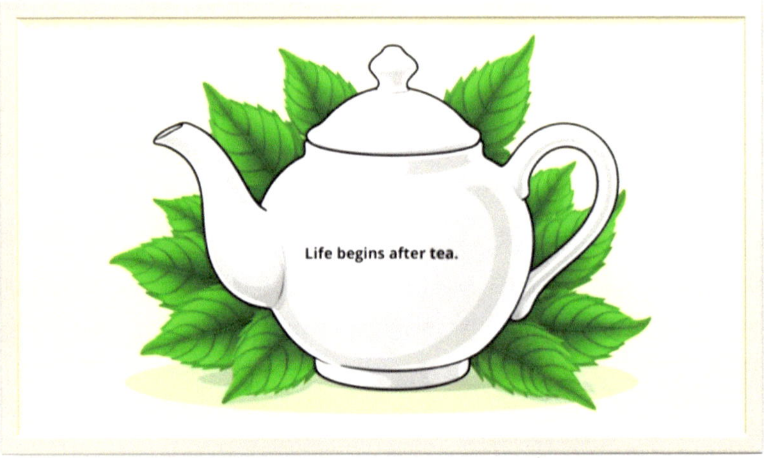
Life begins after tea.

Chapter 11: The Ultimate 21-Day Tea Challenge for Blood Sugar Balance

Balancing blood sugar levels naturally is a goal for many, and incorporating tea into your daily routine can be an easy, enjoyable, and effective way to support this process. Tea is packed with antioxidants, polyphenols, and other bioactive compounds that help regulate glucose levels, improve insulin sensitivity, and reduce inflammation. This **21-Day Tea Challenge** is designed to guide you through a structured plan to harness the power of tea for blood sugar balance.

A STRUCTURED PLAN TO INCORPORATE TEA INTO YOUR DAILY ROUTINE

This challenge follows a simple yet powerful approach:

- You will drink a carefully selected tea every day for 21 days.
- Each tea is paired with a meal or snack to enhance its benefits.
- You will track your progress by journaling how you feel, any changes in energy levels, and your blood sugar readings (if applicable).
- The plan includes a mix of green, herbal,

and spiced teas known for their blood sugar-stabilizing properties.

Let's embark on this journey together and discover how tea can transform your health!

DAILY TEA PAIRINGS WITH MEALS AND SNACKS

To maximize the benefits of tea, we'll pair each tea with a specific meal or snack. Below is your **21-day plan**, divided into three weeks, each with a unique focus.

WEEK 1: STABILIZING BLOOD SUGAR LEVELS

The goal for this week is to introduce teas that help reduce sugar spikes and improve insulin function.

Day 1: Green Tea

Pair with: A protein-rich breakfast (e.g., eggs and avocado toast).

Why? Green tea contains catechins that improve insulin sensitivity and lower blood sugar levels.

Day 2: Cinnamon Tea

Pair with: A mid-morning snack (e.g., almonds and yogurt).

Why? Cinnamon helps slow glucose absorption and enhances insulin function.

Day 3: Ginger Tea

Pair with: A fiber-rich lunch (e.g., quinoa salad with chickpeas).

Why? Ginger has anti-inflammatory properties that support stable blood sugar levels.

Day 4: Hibiscus Tea

Pair with: A light afternoon snack (e.g., nuts and dark chocolate).

Why? Hibiscus tea helps reduce insulin resistance and lowers blood pressure.

Day 5: Fenugreek Tea

Pair with: A high-protein dinner (e.g., grilled salmon and steamed broccoli).

Why? Fenugreek seeds help slow carbohydrate digestion and improve glucose tolerance.

Day 6: Rooibos Tea

Pair with: A bedtime snack (e.g., cottage cheese and walnuts).

Why? Rooibos is caffeine-free and helps reduce stress-related sugar fluctuations.

Day 7: Turmeric Tea

Pair with: Breakfast (e.g., chia pudding with berries).

Why? Turmeric has curcumin, which helps regulate glucose metabolism and combat inflammation.

WEEK 2: IMPROVING INSULIN SENSITIVITY

This week, we focus on teas that enhance insulin function and support metabolism.

Day 8: Oolong Tea

Pair with: A balanced lunch (e.g., grilled chicken with roasted sweet potatoes).

Why? Oolong tea improves fat metabolism and helps regulate blood sugar.

Day 9: Peppermint Tea

Pair with: A light evening meal (e.g., vegetable soup with whole-grain bread).

Why? Peppermint supports digestion and reduces sugar cravings.

Day 10: Chamomile Tea

Pair with: A bedtime routine (e.g., a handful of pumpkin seeds).

Why? Chamomile promotes relaxation and helps regulate glucose levels overnight.

Day 11: Dandelion Root Tea

Pair with: A mid-morning snack (e.g., apple slices with almond butter).

Why? Dandelion root supports liver health and glucose metabolism.

Day 12: Black Tea

Pair with: A high-protein breakfast (e.g., Greek yogurt with flaxseeds).

Why? Black tea polyphenols help slow carbohydrate digestion.

Day 13: Licorice Root Tea

Pair with: A mid-afternoon snack (e.g., hummus with carrots).

Why? Licorice root can help reduce blood sugar spikes after meals.

Day 14: Nettle Tea

Pair with: Dinner (e.g., grilled tofu with quinoa and vegetables).

Why? Nettle tea supports pancreatic function and blood sugar control.

WEEK 3: ENHANCING METABOLISM & LONG-TERM BLOOD SUGAR STABILITY

This final week introduces teas that boost metabolism and provide long-term blood sugar benefits.

Day 15: Matcha Tea

Pair with: A fiber-rich breakfast (e.g., oatmeal with chia seeds).

Why? Matcha has concentrated antioxidants that enhance insulin response.

Day 16: Lemon Balm Tea

Pair with: A light lunch (e.g., avocado and leafy greens salad).

Why? Lemon balm reduces stress and supports glucose metabolism.

Day 17: Clove Tea

Pair with: A mid-morning snack (e.g., mixed nuts and berries).

Why? Cloves have compounds that improve insulin function.

Day 18: Sage Tea

Pair with: A hearty dinner (e.g., grilled chicken with brown rice).

Why? Sage tea helps reduce blood sugar fluctuations.

Day 19: Fennel Tea

Pair with: An afternoon snack (e.g., cottage cheese and pears).

Why? Fennel aids dig

estion and prevents sugar spikes.

Day 20: Ceylon Cinnamon & Green Tea Blend

Pair with: Breakfast (e.g., whole grain toast with peanut butter).

Why? The combination of cinnamon and green tea enhances insulin sensitivity.

Day 21: Your Favorite Blood Sugar-Balancing Tea

Pair with: Any meal of your choice.

Why? By now, you've discovered which tea works best for your body. Keep it as a regular part of your routine!

JOURNALING YOUR PROGRESS AND TRACKING BLOOD SUGAR CHANGES

To get the most out of this challenge, keep a simple daily journal. Each day, note:

- The tea you drank and the meal/snack you paired it with.
- How you felt before and after drinking the tea.
- Any noticeable changes in energy levels, cravings, or digestion.
- If applicable, your blood sugar readings.

By the end of the 21 days, you'll have a clear idea of which teas work best for you and how they impact your body. You may notice improved energy, fewer cravings, better digestion, and more stable blood sugar levels.

YOUR PATH TO LONG-TERM BLOOD SUGAR BALANCE

This **21-Day Tea Challenge** is not just about these three weeks—it's about creating sustainable habits that support your well-being. By continuing to incorporate these teas into your diet, you can maintain stable blood sugar levels, reduce sugar cravings, and enjoy long-term health benefits. Keep exploring new tea blends, listen to your body, and enjoy the journey toward balanced health!

Are you ready to take control of your blood sugar with the power of tea? Let's get started!

Bonus Section: Tea-Based Recipes for Blood Sugar Control

Balancing blood sugar levels is a key factor in maintaining long-term health and overall well-being. Spikes and crashes in blood sugar can lead to fatigue, mood swings, cravings, and even more serious health concerns over time. While diet and exercise play essential roles in blood sugar management, nature offers an incredible array of ingredients that can help regulate glucose levels in a gentle and delicious way. Tea, in particular, is a powerful ally in this quest, providing antioxidants, polyphenols, and other bioactive compounds that support metabolism and insulin sensitivity.

The beauty of tea-based recipes is that they seamlessly combine the benefits of traditional herbal wisdom with modern nutritional science, offering easy-to-make drinks and meals that are both flavorful and functional. From comforting warm beverages to refreshing coolers and nourishing smoothies, each of these recipes has been thoughtfully crafted to incorporate blood sugar-friendly ingredients such as cinnamon, turmeric, hibiscus, and oolong tea. Whether you are looking for a steady source of energy, an anti-inflammatory boost, or a metabolism-enhancing drink, these recipes will provide satisfying solutions to help you feel your best throughout the day.

Enjoy these delicious tea-infused recipes and embrace a healthier, more balanced lifestyle!

CINNAMON GINGER TEA LATTE (WARMING AND BLOOD-SUGAR-FRIENDLY)

This cozy and comforting tea latte is packed with cinnamon and ginger, both of which may help regulate blood sugar levels and improve insulin sensitivity.

Ingredients:

- 1 cup brewed cinnamon tea
- 1/2 teaspoon fresh grated ginger
- 1/2 cup unsweetened almond milk
- 1 teaspoon raw honey or monk fruit sweetener (optional)
- 1/4 teaspoon vanilla extract
- Dash of ground cinnamon for garnish

Instructions:

1. Brew a strong cup of cinnamon tea and add fresh grated ginger.
2. In a small saucepan, heat the almond milk until warm (but not boiling).
3. Blend the tea, almond milk, sweetener, and vanilla extract until frothy.
4. Pour into a mug, sprinkle with ground cinnamon, and enjoy!

MATCHA CHIA PUDDING (A SUPERFOOD BREAKFAST WITH STEADY ENERGY)

This creamy pudding combines matcha and chia seeds for a slow-releasing energy boost while helping to keep blood sugar levels stable.

Ingredients:

- 1 cup unsweetened coconut or almond milk
- 1 tablespoon matcha powder
- 1/4 cup chia seeds
- 1 tablespoon maple syrup or sugar-free sweetener
- 1/2 teaspoon vanilla extract
- Fresh berries or nuts for topping

Instructions:

1. In a bowl, whisk the matcha powder with a small amount of milk until smooth.
2. Add the rest of the milk, chia seeds, sweetener, and vanilla extract. Stir well.
3. Let the mixture sit for 5 minutes, then stir again to prevent clumping.
4. Cover and refrigerate for at least 2 hours or overnight.
5. Serve chilled with fresh berries or nuts on top.

ICED HIBISCUS & MINT COOLER (REFRESHING AND GREAT FOR METABOLISM)

This vibrant iced tea is packed with hibiscus, which is rich in antioxidants and may help lower blood sugar levels.

Ingredients:

- 1 cup brewed hibiscus tea (cooled)
- 5 fresh mint leaves
- 1/2 teaspoon fresh lime juice
- 1 teaspoon raw honey or monk fruit sweetener
- Ice cubes

Instructions:

1. Brew hibiscus tea and let it cool completely.
2. Muddle fresh mint leaves in a glass to release their flavor.
3. Add lime juice and sweetener, then pour in the cooled hibiscus tea.
4. Fill the glass with ice, stir well, and enjoy!

GOLDEN TURMERIC TEA (ANTI-INFLAMMATORY AND BLOOD SUGAR-FRIENDLY)

This soothing tea blend combines turmeric and black pepper, which may help regulate blood sugar and reduce inflammation.

Ingredients:

- 1 cup brewed turmeric tea (or 1 teaspoon fresh grated turmeric in hot water)
- 1/4 teaspoon black pepper
- 1 teaspoon coconut oil or ghee
- 1 teaspoon raw honey or monk fruit sweetener (optional)
- Dash of cinnamon

Instructions:

1. Brew turmeric tea and stir in black pepper.
2. Add coconut oil, honey (if using), and cinnamon.
3. Blend or whisk until creamy and well combined.
4. Pour into a mug and enjoy warm.

OOLONG DETOX SMOOTHIE (METABOLISM-BOOSTING AND DELICIOUS)

This smoothie blends the metabolism-enhancing properties of oolong tea with nutrient-rich ingredients for a balanced, satisfying drink.

Ingredients:

- 1/2 cup brewed oolong tea (cooled)
- 1/2 frozen banana
- 1/4 avocado
- 1/2 cup unsweetened almond milk
- 1 tablespoon flaxseeds

- 1 teaspoon raw honey or monk fruit sweetener (optional)
- Ice cubes (as needed)

Instructions:

1. Brew oolong tea and let it cool completely.
2. In a blender, combine tea, banana, avocado, almond milk, flaxseeds, and sweetener.
3. Blend until smooth, adding ice if desired.
4. Pour into a glass and enjoy immediately.

TEA-INFUSED OATMEAL (FOR BALANCED MORNINGS)

Ingredients:

- 1 cup brewed **cinnamon tea**
- ½ cup rolled oats
- 1 tsp chia seeds
- ½ tsp ground cinnamon
- ½ sliced banana (optional)
- Nuts/seeds for topping

Instructions:

1. Brew **cinnamon tea** and use it instead of water to cook the oats.
2. Add chia seeds and simmer for 3-5 minutes.
3. Top with banana, nuts, and a sprinkle of cinnamon.

Why? This fits **diabetes-friendly guidelines** with

fiber, healthy fats, and **a tea infusion** for extra blood sugar benefits.

GREEN TEA & AVOCADO SMOOTHIE (MID-MORNING ENERGY BOOST)

Ingredients:

- 1 cup chilled **green tea**
- ½ avocado
- ½ cup spinach
- 1 tbsp flaxseeds
- ½ tsp cinnamon
- ½ cup almond milk

Instructions:

1. Blend all ingredients until smooth.
2. Serve chilled and enjoy!

Why? This is a **great way to integrate tea** into meals **without caffeine spikes**.

ROOIBOS & LEMON VINAIGRETTE (FOR SALADS & BOWLS)

Ingredients:

- ¼ cup brewed **rooibos tea**
- 2 tbsp olive oil
- 1 tbsp lemon juice
- 1 tsp Dijon mustard
- ½ tsp garlic powder
- Salt & pepper to taste

Instructions:

1. Whisk ingredients together and use over a **fiber-rich salad**.
2. Store in the fridge for up to 3 days.

Why? Rooibos is naturally caffeine-free and can be a **sugar-free alternative** to commercial salad dressings.

These tea-infused recipes offer a delightful way to support blood sugar balance while savoring rich flavors and wholesome ingredients. Whether you're in the mood for a warm latte, a refreshing iced drink, or a nourishing breakfast, these options make it easy to enjoy the benefits of tea for metabolic health.

A Cup of Wellness – Your Journey Starts Now

Tea is more than a drink. It's a ritual, a moment of pause, a bridge between the past and the present. For centuries, people have turned to tea not just for comfort, but for healing, clarity, and balance. And now, as you reach the end of this book, you hold the same knowledge that countless cultures have cherished for generations—the power of tea to support your body, mind, and health.

REFLECTING ON THE JOURNEY

Think back to when you first picked up this book. Maybe you were curious about whether tea could genuinely help balance blood sugar. Perhaps you've been managing diabetes for years and were looking for a new, natural approach.

Or maybe you're simply a tea lover, eager to deepen your understanding of this ancient, healing beverage. No matter where you started, I hope that by now, you see tea as more than just a warm cup in your hands—you see it as a daily ally in your wellness journey.

We've explored the science behind tea and blood sugar control, the unique compounds that make different teas powerful, and the best ways to prepare and incorporate them into your life.

You now know how green tea's catechins improve insulin sensitivity, how black tea's theaflavins slow carbohydrate absorption, and how herbal infusions like cinnamon, ginger, and hibiscus can naturally support glucose metabolism.

But beyond the research, beyond the technical details, tea has something even greater to offer: a way to slow down, reconnect, and make intentional choices for your health.

WHY TEA IS A LIFELONG COMPANION

I'll be honest with you—I wasn't always a tea purist. I used to think of tea as just another beverage, something to sip absentmindedly while working or watching TV. But the more I learned, the more I experimented, the more I allowed tea to become a ritual, the more I realized its true potential. Tea isn't just about what's in the cup; it's about the experience, the habit, and the connection it fosters with ourselves and the world around us.

Making tea a lifelong habit doesn't mean forcing yourself to drink something you don't enjoy. It means finding the teas that resonate with you, the ones that make you feel good, the ones you look forward to brewing each day. Maybe you love the grassy, slightly sweet taste of a fresh sencha in the morning, or the bold, malty depth of an Assam black tea in the afternoon. Maybe you wind down at night with a floral chamomile blend or a spiced cup of turmeric and cinnamon. There's no right or wrong way to enjoy tea—there's only your way.

MAKING TEA A DAILY RITUAL

One of the most beautiful things about tea is its ability to fit seamlessly into any lifestyle. You don't need to overhaul your entire routine to benefit from its blood sugar-balancing properties. Small, consistent choices can make a lasting impact. Here are a few ways to make tea an effortless part of your daily rhythm:

1. **Start Your Day with Intention**

   Instead of reaching for coffee first thing in the morning, try beginning your day with a cup of green or black tea. Not only does it provide a gentle caffeine boost, but it also sets a mindful tone for the day ahead.

2. **Pair Your Tea with Meals**

   Herbal teas like cinnamon, hibiscus, and ginger can help regulate blood sugar levels when consumed alongside meals. Sipping a warm infusion before or after eating can also aid digestion and prevent glucose spikes.

3. **Use Tea as a Stress Reliever**

   Stress plays a significant role in blood sugar fluctuations. Taking a few minutes to prepare and enjoy a cup of tea can serve as a mini meditation, helping to lower cortisol levels and promote relaxation.

4. **Experiment with Tea Blends**

   One of the most enjoyable parts of a tea journey is discovering new flavors and combinations. Mix and match different herbs and spices to create blends tailored to your needs and preferences.

5. **End Your Day with a Tea Ritual**

   A caffeine-free herbal tea in the evening, like rooibos, chamomile, or valerian root, can signal to your body that it's time to unwind, leading to better sleep and overall balance.

A FINAL WORD OF ENCOURAGEMENT

Changing habits isn't about perfection. It's about small, meaningful steps that add up over time. Maybe you don't drink tea every single day, and that's okay. Maybe some days, you still crave a sugary latte, and that's okay, too. The key is to approach your wellness journey with curiosity and kindness, not restriction and guilt.

Tea is an invitation—an invitation to slow down, to nourish yourself, and to embrace balance. It's a simple act that carries profound benefits, not just for your blood sugar but for your overall well-being. And as you sip your next cup, I hope you remember this: you are in control of your health, and every small, intentional choice brings you closer to vitality and longevity.

So, let this be the beginning of something wonderful. Your journey starts now. May your teacup always be full, your spirit always be nourished, and your health always be thriving.

ABOUT THE BOOK

In a world where diabetes is becoming an increasing concern, *Diabetes & Tea* offers a natural and science-backed approach to managing blood sugar through one of the most ancient and beloved beverages—tea. This book explores the fascinating connection between tea and metabolic health, uncovering the compounds within different tea varieties that may help regulate glucose levels, improve insulin sensitivity, and reduce inflammation.

From green tea's catechins to theaflavins in black tea, and even the benefits of herbal infusions like hibiscus and bitter melon, this book breaks down the best brews for diabetes management. It goes beyond just listing teas—it provides cultural insights, real-life testimonials, and a structured 21-day challenge to incorporate tea into a balanced lifestyle.

With practical guidance on mindful tea rituals, the best brewing methods for maximum benefit, and tips on crafting custom tea blends, *Diabetes & Tea* is more than just a health guide—it's an invitation to embrace a daily habit that can support long-term wellness. Whether you are newly diagnosed, managing diabetes for years, or simply looking for ways to stabilize your blood sugar naturally, this book is your go-to resource for harnessing the power of tea.

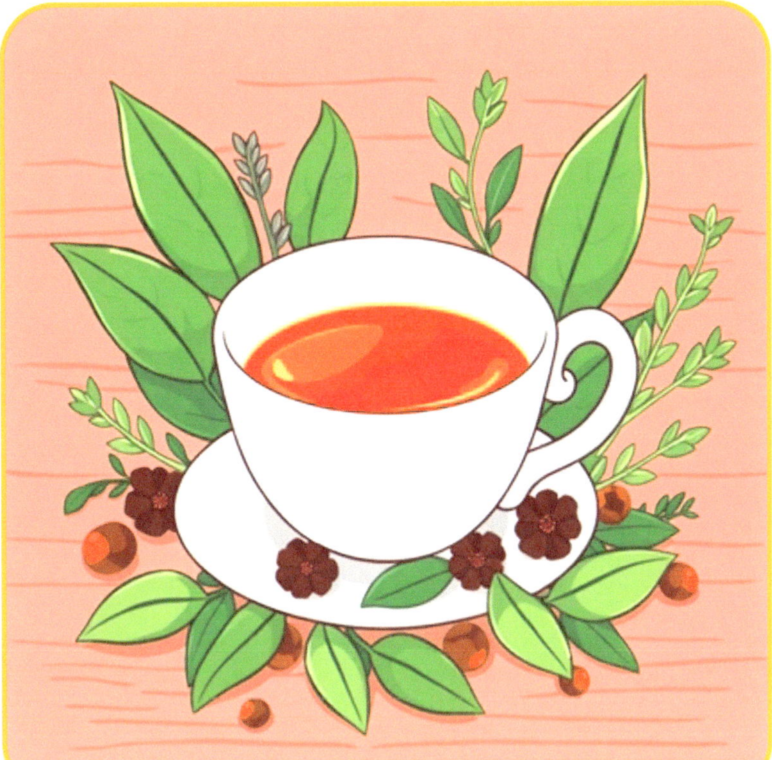

"It's Never Not Teatime!"

Made in the USA
Monee, IL
20 May 2026

50664246R00074